IN THE PRESENCE OF THE MASTERS

IN THE PRESENCE OF THE MASTERS

ROMOLA BUTALIA

Divine Destination
Subsidiary Alliance ~ Motilal Banarsidass Publishing House

Divine Destination

Email: mlbd@mlbd.in • Website: www.mlbd.in

2nd Revised Edition with additional photographs : Delhi, 2022
First Edition : Delhi, 2003

ISBN: 978-93-93214-83-6 (Hardcover)
ISBN: 978-93-93214-90-4 (Paperback)

Printed & Published by
Rajendra P Jain *for*
Motilal Banarsidass Publishing House
A-44, Naraina Industrial Area, Phase I,
New Delhi–110 028 (INDIA)
Email: mlbd@mlbd.in
Website: www.mlbd.in

Whose voice is heard in the silence
Whose breath moves in the stillness
Whose presence is in the void
Who existed before I was born
Who remains when I am gone
Whose effulgence illumines the darkness
Whose shadow falls on the formless
Whose heart is the home of the unattached
Life of my life, Self of my self,
To Thee I offer my All

Contents

List of Photographs

Foreword

One birth is given by your parents, another birth is your own. The first birth is going to end in death. The second birth is the beginning of Eternity: no death—no end—no beginning.

The ultimate goal of earthly life is to experience self-realisation—oneness beyond all change. To be aware, to be awakened is your very first step alone, towards the ultimate "realisation".

Be certain that where everybody is going cannot be the right path. The order of the day is to follow the masses without actually exerting your own intellect, your own consciousness. You have to find a path where none are going. Choose a path that leads you deeper into solitude, into aloneness. Choose a path that is not traditional—not orthodox, basically revolutionary; each step a revolt against all that is past and old.

Only individuals have ever become enlightened. Others become part of a crowd as a Hindu, Christian, Muslim, Jain, Parsi...Crowds never become enlightened. Only individuals who have the courage to be alone are capable of stopping the movement of the mind to settle into their inner innocence.

The deeper you go within yourself, the purer is the source of consciousness that you will find. When you reach the very centre of your being, you reach the centre of the Universe. Then blossoms wisdom and you become a sage.

To experience Liberation, you have to be free from bondage, which is the outcome of your mind. Mind is a conjurer that creates all kinds of illusions: beauty and ugliness, success and failure, riches and poverty. Mind tirelessly creates. Once an idea settles in you, your whole life energy gets consumed in making it a reality. This makes you live in a kind of hypnosis. You can liberate yourself from this hypnosis or bondage. When you become aware that everything is the outcome of mind, be it pain or pleasure, birth or death, and this is seen and known absolutely, the conjurer disappears and what is left is Truth. And that truth liberates you. Realisation brings freedom.

The path to your self is through meditation. Lord Shiva, the ultimate, is constantly in deep meditation, deep penance. He never misses his austerities.

Your consciousness can be Supreme consciousness. The river moves towards the ocean. You will then merge into the whole and not lose yourself. You cannot ever be destroyed in any kind of calamity.

Allow reality to reveal itself. You will come to a state of consciousness where there are no questions left. This state is the answer. There is no answer as such. This Consciousness without any question is the answer, because this consciousness is the most mysterious thing in all of existence, amongst all the mysteries of life.

Sankalpit Yoga is the science of creation. Like everything in nature, Gyana (knowledge) has come through Sankalpa. Sankalpit Yoga does not belong to anyone in particular, nor is it registered by any organisation. It belongs to all those who want to practice it. There is no one to command you. There is no market for it to be sold in. There is no bondage. There are no milestones. You have to walk away from the bridge, away from the master.

Mahayogi Pilot Baba
Mahamandaleshwar, Juna Akhara,
Talla Gethia,
Nainital-263 130 (Himalayas)

ENLIGHTENED MASTERS

CHAPTER 1

Sacred Spaces

"Wherefrom do all these worlds come?
They come from space.
All beings arise from space, and into space they return;
Space is indeed their beginning,
And space is their final end."

— *Chandogya Upanishad*

In 1985, as I climbed the last of the steps up the hill from our house to the main road in Almora, where we lived at the time, I saw a freshly painted sign that stated simply, 'Pilot Baba'. It registered in my consciousness. I knew that when I came across the name again, I would remember where I had first learnt of it. It was inevitable that I would hear it many times since.

We lived at Bright End Corner, adjacent to the Rama Krishna Mission Ashram. Being neighbours, we were friendly with the *sadhus* living there, particularly Swami Ishanandaji, who was the Head Swamiji. He used to come daily to borrow our newspaper as his reached the next day. He would invariably join us for a cup of coffee. Sometimes he would cook *upma* for us and bring it over. We were always invited for a meal on special occasions like the birthday celebrations of Rama Krishna Paramhansa, Swami Vivekananda and Sarada Ma.

Ishanandaji would invite us over to meet his close friends. Once he called me to meet an aged *sannyasi* who was a direct disciple of Sarada Ma. He asked me about my ancestral lineage. My grandfather, Nabajiban Banerji, who passed away when I was five, was a doctor. During his college days, he would skip lunch to save money to pay a friend's college fees. Later, he spent all the money he earned on running a hospital where people could avail free treatment. He was regarded as an eccentric by the worldly, because he would wear shorts, believing that the cloth so saved could be of use to someone else.

When I mentioned my grandfather's name, the old *sadhu* expressed great joy and blessed me. "Before we had built our own hospital, Nabajiban Babu told us that he would be happy to give whatever medical attention any of us needed. I often wondered where his descendants are."

Swami Ishanandaji was always generous with his blessings. He allowed me complete access to the library built specifically for *sadhus* in retreat. I had the opportunity to read rare books I had not come across elsewhere. He often used to tell me to write. I would laugh and say, "What should I write about?" He would reply, "What you have read and understood." I took it lightly. I had always read for my own enjoyment and understanding.

The last time I met him, he had made me promise that I would write an article on any topic I wanted. "If for nothing else, because I have asked it of you," he had said. My first published travelogue, which led me to journalism, was about our trek to Pindari glacier. In it I had written:

"For the better part of three years I had watched the snow-capped peaks from afar: glistening as the first rays of sunlight touched them; remote and majestic with wisps of clouds playing hide-and-seek later in the morning; hidden from view by a myriad clouds as the day progressed; golden in the dying sunlight; silver-streaked by moonlight.

"The moods of the seasons played different tunes: in winter they stood totally covered by snow, untouched; in spring they whispered promises of times to come, in summer they hid from the view of curious onlookers; in monsoons they were speckled with every hue of the rainbow; and in autumn they prepared to remain aloof. Then, one day they beckoned to come closer and we were on our way to the Pindari glacier."

About one of the many travellers we had met on the path, I had written: "We met a Himalayan sage, walking bare-bodied in the snow, once a familiar, well-loved and deeply revered *sadhu* of these hills, now very rarely seen. He walked carrying nothing, not even his name, and he left behind nothing, not even his footprints, and in passing he gave me a koan I know will take a lifetime to fathom."

At Almora, there were several *sadhus* living in the nearby hills with whom we were very friendly. If an unknown *sadhu* came by, he was always offered food. Once a particular mendicant mentioned that he was going on a pilgrimage to the higher Himalayas and needed something warm to wear. On leaving, he gave a *rudraksha* in blessing saying, "If you ever want anything, hold this *rudraksha* in your hand, and wish for what you want, and your wish will come true." In turn, I had said to the *sadhu* as he left, "I cannot bless you, but my best wishes go with you that you may live in awareness of God." He replied, "*Yeh unhi ki lila hai.*" (This world is His play of consciousness).

Our close friend and neighbour, known as Mataji to everyone in the vicinity, had lived in Benares at her *guru's ashram* for 17 years before she shifted to Almora, when her *guru* left his mortal body. We met her daily. If I did not visit her during the day, she would come across to our house in the evening. Shivaji, a young renunciate, had been given permission by his *guru* to stay with her. He had been instructed not to go to the home of a householder except to ask for alms. Shivaji presumed his *guru* would have permitted his coming to our house with her.

After an immensely enjoyable evening spent together over dinner, the next morning I heard the mendicant's greeting at the door, '*Om Namoh Narayana*'. Acknowledging the ascetic standing at the door, I went to fetch some rice that I offered him. He gave me ashes from his *dhuni* as a blessing before he left. At the time, as part of his *tapasya,* Shivaji walked barefoot. Our four-year-old son, Siddhartha discreetly suggested that I give him slippers. I gave Siddhartha a somewhat hurried explanation, that since he was looking for God, he did not want to wear slippers. Siddhartha asked, "You cannot look for God in slippers?"

Later, we visited Shivaji while he was staying with his *guru*, Kali Baba, under a tree near Baijnath. Shivaji was a little anxious whether Kali Baba would baulk at his Westernised friends. Kali Baba welcomed us with warmth and grace and invited us to share a simple meal of rice and chutney, exquisitely cooked on a log fire under the blue Himalayan skies. We shared a lovely afternoon of laughter and conversation with him. He said, "I live at Vaikunth's door (the abode of Vishnu). I recognise who you are." A few hours later when we were leaving, I was startled to see tears in his eyes. I folded my hands in humble acknowledgement.

At the time, we used to frequent Tara's teashop at Kasar Devi. One day invited for dinner at Tara's home, we saw a photograph of him with Pilot Baba. Tara told us that a few years earlier, Pilot Baba had taken *sthal samadhi*, and he had kept vigil at the site for the seven days he had been underground. Later still, we read in the newspapers that Pilot Baba had taken *jal samadhi* somewhere.

One day my husband, Rajiv, called from his office, "Would you like to meet Pilot Baba? We have been invited to dinner by someone whose house he is visiting."

I had heard that Pilot Baba got his name from having been a Wing Commander in the Indian Air Force. Rumour had it that during a particular mission, his plane was spiralling downwards to sure disaster when he had been saved. In 1972, he renounced the world. When I met him, I did not ask him about his past, being aware that a sannyasi forsakes his past in ritual renunciation. I did not enquire about reports of his ability to withhold his breathing for several days during *jal* and *sthal samadhi*. Somehow 'miracles' had never fascinated me.

As a special concession from the tradition of our hosts, I was invited to join the men for dinner. Immediately after Pilot Baba took his first mouthful, he turned to me and it was the pilot, clad in saffron, who emerged to apologise, "I am sorry I had not noticed that you had not started eating." His deep and abiding respect for women is something I had occasion to witness many times since.

That evening I asked Pilot Baba, "What is your normal state of consciousness?" I was keen to know whether people could maintain a meditative state of consciousness while dealing with the everyday world. I wanted to be allowed a glimpse of that state. However, for that I had to wait a few years.

CHAPTER 2

Spiritual Awakening

"He is seen in Nature
In the wonder of a flash of lightning.
He comes to the soul
In the wonder of a flash of vision."

— *Kena Upanishad*

In 1989, in the rarefied atmosphere of the higher Himalayas, in a valley close to the Pindari glacier, we noticed a small cave, painted with the words, 'Pilot Baba'. Two days later, on our way back from our trek to Pindari glacier, we had stopped for the night at the village of Khati, where we overheard that Pilot Baba was soon arriving.

As dusk fell, he arrived with several other *sadhus*, having trekked the hard 20 km distance from Song to the tiny village of Khati, where legend has it that the descendants of those who had sheltered the Pandavas lived. Along with the entire village, and several of the trekkers, we went to the room where they sat. We looked around the room where three saffron-clad *yogis* of indeterminate age were seated, not recognising Pilot Baba from our earlier meeting. He announced, "I am Pilot Baba. I cut my hair at the recent *Kumbh*." People came seeking *darshan*, prostrating themselves before him. Most of the trekkers came out of curiosity. Soon everyone had left but we remained awhile in conversation.

Along with them was Keiko Aikawa, who would be staying secluded for several days in a cave at Pindari, for which she was preparing herself. One of the sages teasingly remarked that all the villagers were coming to pay their respects to Pilot Baba, that he himself had been that way as many times and more, but they did not come to him. Keiko Mata said, "Maybe they do not see you. Maybe you are invisible." At the time we laughed at the statement.

Hearing me speak to Pilot Baba in English, the *yogi* turned and said to me, "Convent *mein pareh ho.*" (You have studied in a convent). I nodded and explained that being Bengali, my Hindi was very weak. He spoke to me affectionately in Bengali. Turning to 7-year-old Siddhartha, he conversed with him, while Rajiv and I talked to Pilot Baba. He called our attention with, "Listen to what this boy is saying."

He asked Siddhartha, "Will you take me to school with you?"

Siddhartha nodded.

He asked, "Will you introduce me to your friends as your friend?"

Siddhartha again nodded.

The yogi laughed and taking Siddhartha on his lap, hugged him. Siddhartha, who had lived in Almora between the ages of two and five, was very used to seeing *sadhus* and did not differentiate between them and anyone else. He was also used to having friends of varied ages. He grew up in an atmosphere where he, and the other children nearby, would scamper freely around the hillside, going across to meet whomever they chose. He was very friendly with all the neighbours, including the *sadhus* at the Rama Krishna Mission Ashram next door.

Siddhartha's childhood was spent in sacred spaces amongst many different people from all of whom he received much love. He regarded all of them as his friends. Now meeting this unknown *yogi*, he could readily accept him as just another friend and saw no reason to think that he could not be introduced as one.

Later, standing outdoors, chatting with one of the other *sadhus* accompanying Pilot Baba, we enquired about the identity of this *yogi.* We were told, "He is Hariakhan Baba. He is Kripacharya of the Mahabharata." When Pilot Baba stepped out, we put the same question to him and he replied, without offering any explanation, "He is Gorakh Baba."

After dinner, wanting to discuss spiritual matters, we requested permission to spend a little more time with them. It was bitterly cold. Siddhartha was fast asleep, exhausted from the trekking. Rajiv carried him and sat with him in his lap. Gorakh Baba handed me a large *rajbhog* (sweetmeat) and pointing to Rajiv said, "50-50."

The minutes turned to hours as we talked about the Mind, about cycles of birth and death, about the spiritual path. Pilot Baba asked me why I am doing what I am doing with my life. I answered, "Because I enjoy it." Wanting to clarify my interpretation of death experience and of re-birth, I asked him if what I believed could indeed be the truth. He said, "it is 100 per cent true."

I asked him where I stood and where I had to go. Repeating what I had said at different points of our conversation, he said, "You enjoy, you know and you believe. You have nowhere to go. You will never have a *guru.* Seek the Truth in your experiences of life from everyone you meet."

While he talked, it seemed to me that he spelt out the milestones I would cross as I would walk ahead. I listened intently. Every time I have reached the hard-won understanding I sought, I knew he had given me a glimpse of it in sharing his wisdom and learning.

As we sat talking, Gorakh Baba was meditating silently. Hearing him utter a sound that came from the very depths of his being, I apologized that we had stayed too long and had disturbed him. Pilot Baba quickly reassured us, "No one is disturbed by conversation like this."

Early the next morning, as we prepared to set out for the day's trek, I stopped at their door to say goodbye to both of them. Gorakh Baba said, "Life is a question. Solve it."

I bowed my head in acceptance of the koan. He said,

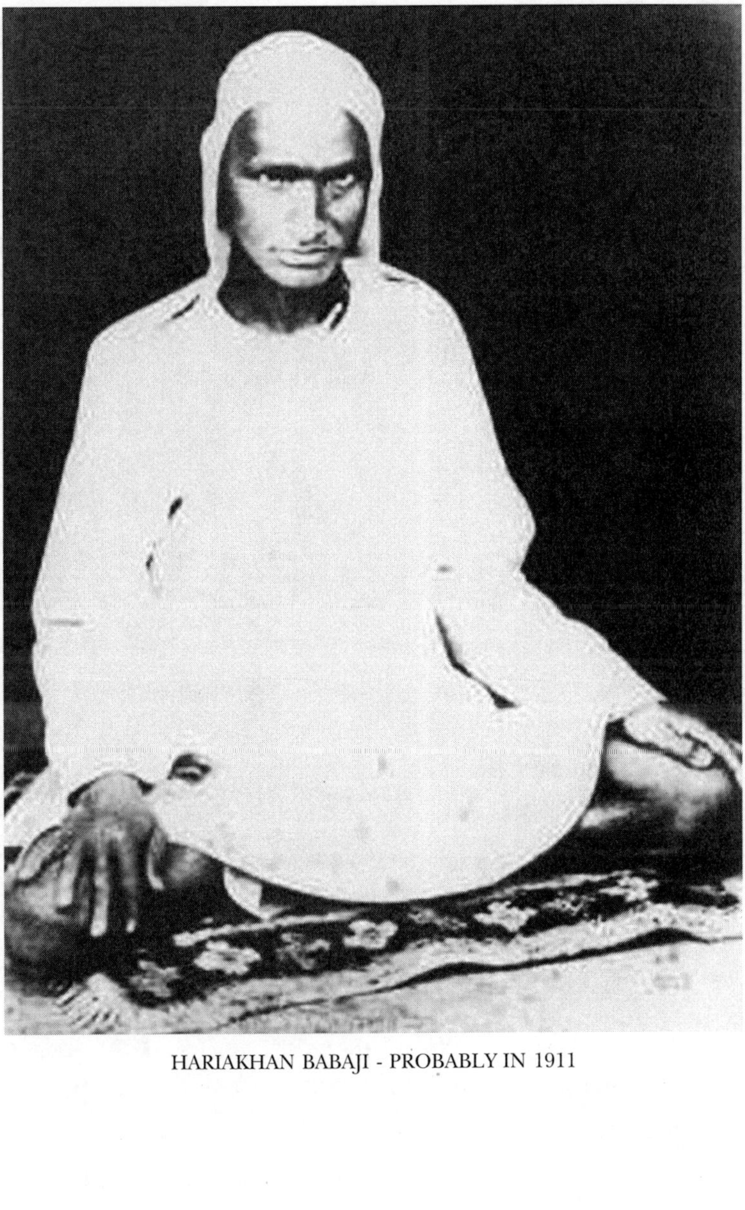

HARIAKHAN BABAJI - PROBABLY IN 1911

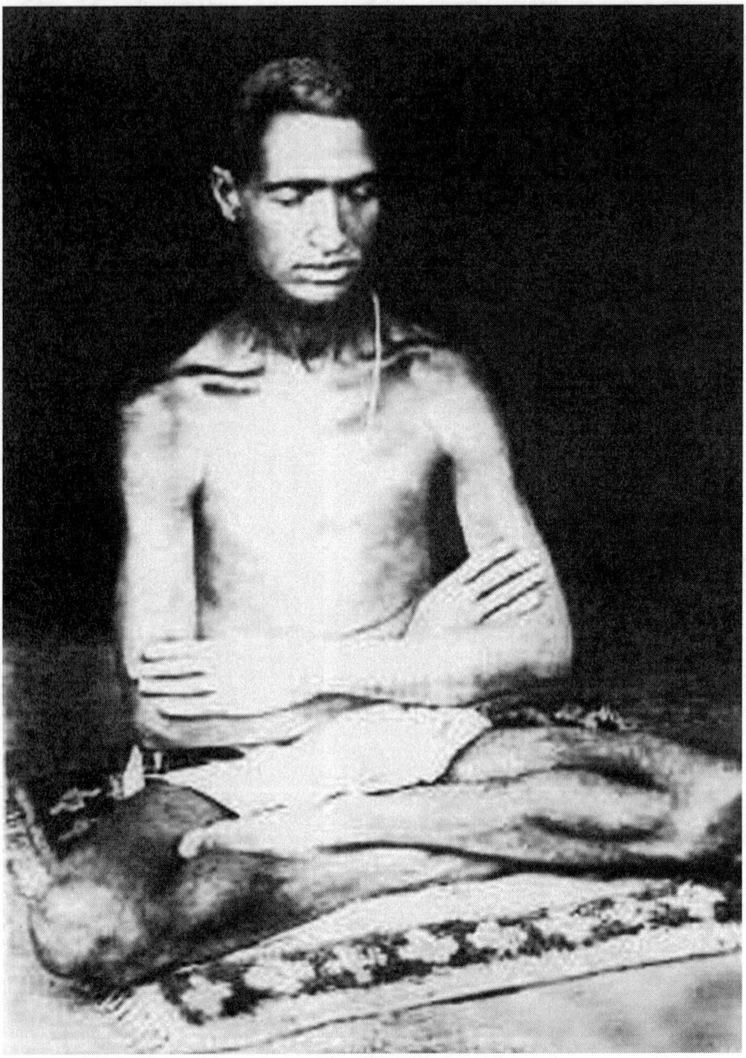

HARIAKHAN BABAJI - PHOTO TAKEN AT THE SAME TIME

"Remember that," and repeated himself, "Life is a question. Solve it." Over the years, in my attempt to solve it, I meditated with my life itself.

On our way back from Pindari glacier, we stopped at Almora to meet several of our friends who still lived there. We recounted the experiences of our trek to Dr. Tim Rees, who had spent some fifteen years in a Zen monastery in Japan and later joined Sri Aurobindo's Ashram at Pondicherry. During the years we had lived in Almora, he would visit us frequently. He said he could not place Gorakh Baba, but expressed surprise that we had met Hariakhan Baba, informing us that he is no longer in his mortal body.

Mashima was not immediately familiar with the names. About Rees' comment she added, "Anything is possible. There are sages who are *videhi.* They move in their astral forms and can materialise and dematerialise their bodies. My *guru* knew many of them. I have heard there is a place in the Himalayas, sometimes referred to as 'Gyanganj'. You cannot reach there except in your astral body, or unless you are taken there by an adept. A disciple of my master had been there. Many advanced disciples practice different yogic sciences there."

We were not much wiser about who Gorakh Baba was. The notion of having or moving in one's astral body did not arouse much curiosity. We had read accounts of such feats in Yogananda Paramhansa's *Autobiography of a Yogi.*

A few years later on a trek to Gaumukh, the source of the Ganga, I met an old *sadhu.* I enquired if Pilot Baba or Gorakh Baba had crossed that way. He replied that Pilot Baba had not been there recently and Gorakh Baba cannot be seen. I said that we had met Gorakh Baba a few years earlier. He folded his hands in acknowledgement and said, "Then you have been blessed by him."

One day, absorbed in reading *Living with the Himalayan Masters,* I saw an obviously old photograph captioned

Hariakhan Baba. I thought it was the same person we had met. Hiding the caption, I showed the picture to Rajiv. He confirmed that it looked like Gorakh Baba. I did the same with Siddhartha, who said, "We met him on the way to Pindari."

Later I learnt that the picture was supposed to have been taken in 1911, by a photographer, Sorabji, who had taken two photographs of him at the time. The story goes that when the reel was developed, one photograph depicted him with a robe and cap, and the other showed him without them.

Sometimes I would read references to Guru Gorakh Nath or Mahavtar Baba or Hariakhan Baba. I did not attempt to unravel the puzzle of who he is, but focused more on the koan he had given me.

In recent years, it seemed to me that I had walked a long way without meeting the sages who once crossed my path frequently, each of whom gave me, in passing, a glimpse of their own realisation. I had been content to walk on. I had wondered where Pilot Baba now is, but I had not actively sought to meet him, as I had not sought any of the experiences of my life, sure that my destiny awaited me and I would reach it, if I were free of the search for it.

One day someone wrote to me about their trekking experiences. I read the name Pilot Baba and started. Was it the writing on the wall again? Was it time for another meeting then?

Chapter 3

Mahayogi Kapil Advait

"I know that Spirit whose infinity is in all,
Who is ever one beyond time.
I know the Spirit
Whom the lovers of Brahman call eternal,
Beyond the birth and rebirth of life."

— *Svetasvatara Upanishad*

Mahayogi Kapil Advait is popularly known as Pilot Baba. His life is well recorded. Pilot Baba describes his own childhood as carefree and innocent, his adolescence as an age of angst and daring. His youth was a mixture of high adventure and patriotic idealism. Soon there was a conflict between the call of worldly values and youthful dreams with the path of spiritual renunciation.

At frequent intervals throughout his life, he was visited by Hari Baba, who first met and played with him as a child outside his ancestral home in Bihar. Whenever his mother spotted him playing with the *yogi*, she felt uneasy about it. Pilot Baba says, "Her motherly instincts always warned her whenever she saw me in the company of the Baba. Even a casual reference to my growing fondness for him used to upset her greatly. She nursed secret fears that Baba would take me away from her one day. Despite all her caution, events happened according to Baba's wishes".

Hari Baba regularly visited him at Darjeeling where he went to school, on his travels abroad, at other unexpected times and places. He was always there when his advice or protection was needed.

One day, in the early hours of the morning, he sat with friends at Tiger Top enjoying the beauty of the rising sun. Perched on a rock, he began to muse philosophically about life and death. Hari Baba joined the pensive gathering. Unable to contain the tumult that raged within him, he spoke to Baba candidly. "Baba, can one escape from the spectre of death and live fearlessly? I feel as though I am continuously hounded by death. I want to run away from myself and seek refuge in the distant hills, which seem to be devoid of any sign of life."

His outburst stunned his friends. Baba looked at his face with a penetrating glance, smiled and said, "Penance in the Himalayan caves is the answer to your query. These caves are untouched by the fear which is constantly pursuing you."

He explained, "Man's *karmas* instil these fears. *Karmas* give birth to a sequence of incidents, which finally culminate in man's destruction. But man, if he seriously wills, can keep death at bay. He must first learn to destroy his *samskaras*, and should also escape from the birth of new *samskaras*. *Tapasya* is the only medium which can offer total deliverance from worldly fetters."

Pilot Baba says, "The roots of fear were so deep that Baba's illuminating words were not enough. Baba read my mind like an open book. His next move was totally unexpected. He gave me a big push and I went hurtling down into the depths of a ravine. Baba appeared cool, almost unconcerned with the accident. My friends were infuriated with his nonchalance and began to chase him, but were unable to catch the racing figure of Baba.

"While I was hurtling downwards, two invisible mysterious hands supported me. Baba took off into the air and began to fly like a winged person right over my falling figure. He finally swooped down and prevented me from dashing myself against the rocky ground. My clothes were in tatters, but surprisingly, I did not have a single scratch on my body. Baba brought me back safe and sound to my friends. Despite the ordeal that I had gone through, I was laughing and in high spirits. Baba was also laughing with me.

"He gave us some fruits, took the customary fee of Rs 2 that he always collected from me and departed from the scene. This seemingly miraculous escape left a deep imprint on everyone's mind. I was in a dream-like state and secretly toyed with the idea of *tapasya* and asceticism."

One day when he was visiting Elephant's Fall at Shillong, he settled comfortably on a rock that faced the waterfall. The instant his body touched the rocky seat, he went into a dream-like state. The shower of gentle droplets from the cascading waterfall did not disturb his trance. A vision began to unfold in which he saw himself moving in the narrow pathways of a mountainous region. There was a strange sense of familiarity about the place and the people. He came out of his trance with the ear-splitting sound of an explosion from a small plane, which burst into flames and fell on the nearby trees.

Attempting to locate the burnt remains of the plane, he could not see anything. Pilot Baba says, "Everything that had occurred belonged to the world of dreams. It was a unique experience, which cannot be comprehended by those who dwell in the physical-sensory plane. Following the mystical experience, a new urge forced me to walk to the forests. All the pathways of the forests appeared familiar to me and emboldened by the sense of familiarly, I continued to tread ahead. The roads took me to a habitation, which again, had a strange familiarity about it. I felt as though I had often trudged through these lanes."

Pilot Baba continues, "I went to a cluster of shops and enquired about some people in the Khasi dialect spoken there. I was amazed at my own fluency in an alien tongue. The people I had enquired about were long dead. Only a couple of very old men could throw some light on my queries.

"One of them spoke to me, 'the nature of your vision is purely mystical. You must immediately forewarn the authorities that no plane should fly over this area for it will meet a fiery end. Your vision has foretold a future incident'. We started walking back together. After a short silence, the old man said, 'Can you give me Rs. 2?' Immediately I discerned his identity. He was my old acquaintance, Hari Baba."

Sobered by this divine phenomenon, he returned to camp and forewarned the concerned authorities about the future accident. People laughed at him and declared him a victim of hallucinations. He tried his best to avert the disaster but no one paid the least attention to his precognition. The disaster did occur according to his vision and the unfortunate pilot died a tragic death.

One day, overcome with nostalgia, he applied for leave. Early one morning, brooding over the rejection of his leave application, on impulse, he took out his jeep and started driving towards town through the thick fog. Due to poor visibility and bad driving, his jeep collided against a bridge, and began to roll backwards. It fell into a deep gorge.

Pilot Baba describes the incident, "I could feel myself falling into the dangerous depths of the ravine. Before I met a sure ghastly death, a miracle occurred. A pair of invisible hands caught me and gently brought me back to the bridge. I was too stunned to react, so I could not even thank my unknown rescuer. The incident had created a stir amidst onlookers to the accident. Everyone began to congratulate me at my good fortune. Some talked about an unknown *sadhu* who had rescued me. His identity could not be ascertained by anyone and his appearance remained a mystery. Outwardly I remained quiet, but inwardly I knew the answer to this riddle."

Describing another incident, Pilot Baba says, "Once, while I was flying over NEFA, my plane began to lose height. Despite my best efforts, I could not control the plane. I could have ejected out of the plane but decided against it. The mountains, like angry giants, loomed closer as an air crash seemed imminent. I made one final effort to take the plane towards the distant river, but did not succeed. All the controls had stopped functioning so any attempt to avert the disaster appeared impossible. I braced myself for the final confrontation. The yawning mountains echoed one word only: death.

"At that instant, again, a miracle occurred and the falling plane began to gain height. I was mystified by this phenomenon. All the controls began to function normally. Unbelievable as it may sound, the only significant difference was that a mysterious *yogi* landed the plane. Before it could come to a halt, the *yogi* vanished without a word. I took the plane near the hangar and safely grounded it. The officials at the control room had given up all hopes of my survival when they could not trace my plane on the radar.

"When my plane appeared on the screen everyone gasped in amazement. Till date this remains one of many aviation mysteries. I am the sole witness to the circumstances that led to this impending disaster and of the saviour who brought me back from the doors of death. Why did this *yogi* help me at a critical juncture in my life? I was weighed down by this thought. I pondered the question but came to no logical conclusion."

Later, when a well-dressed man came to him while he was with his friends at Nashik and requested him for Rs 2, he recognized him instantly. Soon the man returned, dressed in saffron, and hurried away waving the Rs 2 he had been given, while the young pilot was left wanting to ask him many questions. Analysing this, he realized that it was time to forsake the clothes he wore and don the garb of a renunciate.

As a pilot, he was a recipient of two gallantry awards. He was attached to the VIP squad where he was assigned to duty with Indira Gandhi, Prime Minister of India, at the time. He requested permission to be discharged from the Air Force because of his desire to renounce the world. She refused permission. Subsequently assigned to duty with Zakir Hussain, President of India, he explained his predicament, and had his discharge papers signed by him.

Two days later, Zakir Hussain passed away. Indira Gandhi, on hearing that he was leaving the Air Force said, "I would not have relieved you of duty. The papers are already signed and there is now no way to change that fact."

Feelings of detachment overpowered him and he renounced the world willingly. Thereafter he roamed around desperately seeking the *guru* who had awakened his spirituality. At intervals he would return to a familiar world of friends and distractions. A fleeting glimpse of Hari Baba at the Shiva Ratri Mela at Pashupatinath Temple in Kathmandu left him frantically hunting for his *guru* again.

One day, forsaking everything, he walked on the banks of the Narayani with the sole aim of finding Hari Baba. When he found a suitable rock in the solitude of dense forests, he took off his clothes and sat in a posture of penance. Tired and worn out, just before he fell asleep, he sighted Hari Baba carrying a small bundle of twigs and an axe. Seemingly hypnotised by his presence, he felt he was being dragged in a particular direction. Pilot Baba says, "Within no time we were face to face with a celestial looking *yogi*."

The *yogi* welcomed them both, saying, "Hari Baba, you have finally accomplished your mission." Turning towards Pilot Baba, he said, "We have been waiting for you for millennia. It is very difficult to break the traditional bondage of the physical world. Hari has been pursuing you through several incarnations. This path is strewn with many obstacles. When consciousness of the soul dawns upon a man, his mind begins to court *vairagya* or renunciation. It is very difficult to resurrect these s*amskaras* and mitigate *prarabdh* karma. After undergoing many austerities, a person beholds the inner light. Thereafter, a *jeeva* becomes alone and surrenders himself totally to this inner light. The state of self-cognition follows soon, which finally culminates in divine cognition. Hari Baba's relationship with you is many incarnations old. I, too, have awaited your coming.

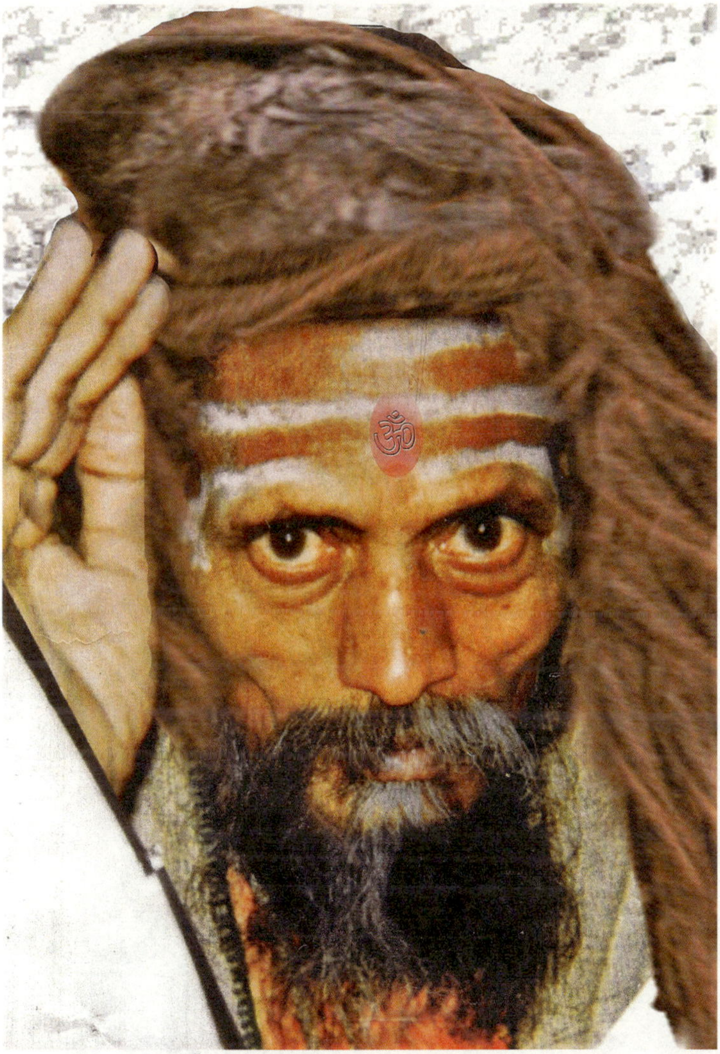

HARI BABA - PILOT BABAJI'S GURU

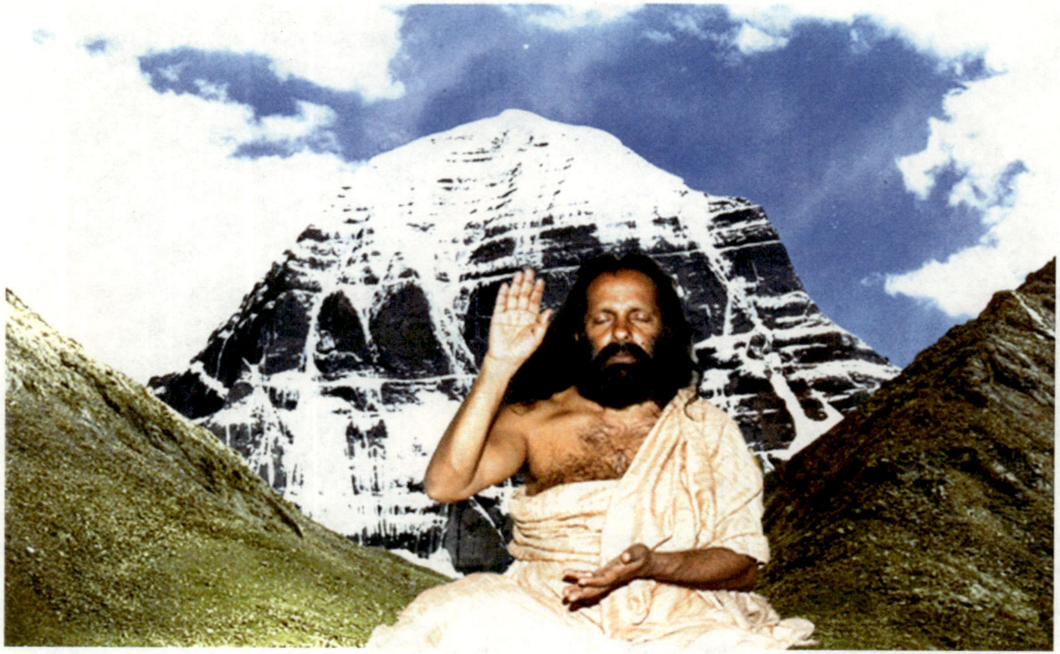

PILOT BABAJI - IN THE HIMALAYAS

Kapil, immerse yourself totally in the infinite ocean of spiritualism and enjoy divine bliss. A man who is caught in the web of life and death does not have time to delve in spiritual ecstasy."

So began the spiritual transformation that caused a successful young pilot to renounce the world and, in time, become a *mahayogi.*

Pilot Baba has given his blessings to many and has readily shared his knowledge and wisdom with seekers. He represents human ability to transcend the world and yet live ithin its folds, to go beyond birth and death. The messages I have heard him give are as varied as the different words he uses to convey them. He has repeatedly said, "I want to bring them suffering, so they may be forced to seek deliverance."

I have watched his reactions in different circumstances. I have seen him deal with hundreds of people. I have witnessed a human being of many facets who can transcend his own being to move with ease in different realms of living. I recognize in him a master who gives of himself to the world. He does not seek to be deified. He always says, "The master is only a bridge. Don't worship the master. The master is not god." He also says, "Realisation cannot be given to another. You have to realise yourself."

Pilot Baba is a familiar being I recognize well. I have seen his human face as I have seen the *yogi* and the *mahayogi.* His knowledge, understanding and wisdom are infinite indeed for he has known the *Brahmanda* beyond and can move in many different spaces. In recent times, every breath he has taken has been dedicated to sharing his energy with others. I salute him for being a perfect teacher.

CHAPTER 4

Pieces of a Puzzle

Gorakh Nath:
"Which is the root and which is the branch?
Who is the guru and who the disciple;
With what essence can one go about alone?"
Matsyendra Nath:
"Mind is the root and vital breath is the branch;
The word is the guru and attention is the disciple.
With the essence called deliverance,
Gorakh Nath wanders about, himself in himself."

— *Gorakhbodh*

Roy Eugene Davis, a direct disciple of Yogananda Paramhansa wrote in his book, *The Kriya Yoga Way of Soul Liberation,* that an illumined master known as Babaji is acknowledged as the spiritual head of the current era Kriya Yoga tradition. Davis wrote, "Little is known about this legendary personage because he prefers to work from behind the scenes, communicating directly with advanced disciples. Babaji has been in his present body for several centuries and is known by different names in different places."

There are innumerable stories about Babaji, though there are no records of when he was born, where he hails from, or any historical facts associated with events in his life. There are many legends about him that place him as living in different centuries and varied places.

He is said to have initiated Lahiri Mahashaya in 1861, and later met his disciple, Sri Yukteshwar who was Yoganandaji's *guru.* Davis wrote, "Several close disciples of Lahiri Mahashaya also had personal contact with Babaji over the years in the Himalayas or when the master would visit them in subtle form. Babaji can appear to persons in his light body and he can materialise and dematerialise his physical body at will."

Davis mentions, "It is said about Baba Gorakh Nath that he could 'ride the air' as he would sometimes quickly traverse large distances. He was known to appear at two or more places at the same time."

Pilot Baba recalls the first time he met Gorakh Baba. One night at Baljuriya Peak, Pilot Baba noticed a ray of light pierce the blanket of fog. Gradually the figure of a tall lanky man in yellow robes became discernible. For sometime he seemingly floated through the air before he began to descend to the icy ground. Walking towards Pilot Baba, he was soon sitting next to him. His arrival startled Pilot Baba because everything had happened in such rapid succession. Paying his respects to the celestial being, Pilot Baba looked at him inquiringly. When he remained unresponsive, Pilot Baba elected to lie on the icy bed and watch the glittering stars and planets.

After a brief lull, the *Mahatma* asked, "Aren't you surprised at my arrival? Why this sudden interest in the skies?" In a calm voice Pilot Baba replied, "Sir, you have come of your own will, and will also leave of your own will. Initially, I had many questions to ask, but your apparent disinterest discouraged me. I had no option but to ask the skies instead. I was not surprised because many *Mahatmas* often travel via the air route. Their movements are controlled by their will power. Their powers are a result of their *samskaras.* Since I cannot have similar *samskaras,* I should not unnecessarily show interest in such superhuman feats. Since you are a divine *purush,* I look upon you with great reverence. I know that your *karmas* cannot help me and that I have to enjoy the fruits of my own *karmas.* I know that my accidental meeting with you is the result of my *samskaras.*"

Hearing Pilot Baba speak, the enlightened being smiled and gently drew him closer. Pilot Baba looked closely at his quiet, unassuming face. He says, "He seemed quite familiar, but I could not recollect where and when I had seen him."

The afternoon I spoke to Pilot Baba of Gorakh Baba, during our prolonged conversation, he looked towards the open door and said, "You were talking of Gorakh Baba, he is here." Within a minute or two, as I looked expectantly, Gorakh Baba took long strides into the room. When I had last met him in the cold of Khati 12 years ago, Gorakh Baba had worn a single cloth. This time when he came, he was wearing a full-sleeved robe and had a muffler on his head as though he had just stepped down to the hot and dusty plains of India from the bitter cold of the lofty heights of the Himalayas.

Davis wrote, "Public ceremonies were encouraged for the welfare of the people and to encourage a harmonious relationship with the forces of nature." At Bharatpur, where I met him in October 2001, I heard Gorakh Baba mention to Pilot Baba that since he had been invited for a *yagna*, it was imperative that he come. He attended the *yagna* on the first day, sitting beside Pilot Baba throughout and participating in the entire proceedings.

Pandit Rajmani Tigunait wrote, "Sages of Guru Gorakh Nath's calibre are literally the word of God in flesh. At the behest of his master, this immortal *yogi* has been guiding sincere aspirants for more than a millennium. Even today we hear occasional reports from those who have met him and received guidance from him."

My own impressions of him were of a warm, immensely caring human being. Perpetually absorbed in deep meditation, he glanced around him occasionally, almost as though his vision was of a different space. When I first met him, at my initial glance I saw a perfect *yogi*. With a stern and serious disposition, distant and aloof, he was completely still, a perpetual witness without any vibrations. Soon I noticed a gentle, playful, happy child in his interactions with Siddhartha. He was the immortal master when his blessing came in words of eternal wisdom. I saw a friend in his parting words, "I will talk to you again." I recognized him as someone very familiar whom I have always known.

CHAPTER 5

Legends of Gorakh Nath

"Oh life-giving sun, offspring of the Lord of creation,
Solitary seer of heaven!
Spread thy light and withdraw thy blinding splendour
That I might behold thy radiant form:
That Spirit far away within thee is my own inmost Spirit"

— *Isha Upanishad*

Pandit Rajmani Tigunait referred to the divine birth of Guru Gorakh Nath in his book, *From Death to Birth.* He wrote, "the eternal sage Narayana himself walks in the flesh in the form of Matsyendra Nath. Realising the depth of human ignorance and misery he resolved to help the human race through a beloved disciple who had already left his body and become one with universal consciousness."

Among the many stories that abound, legend has it that as the eternal sage Matsyendra Nath walked through a village, he stopped at a house where he was given a meal. Blessing the woman who gave it, he said he would grant her any wish she had. When she mentioned that she was barren, he gave her some ash from the fire pit and told her to eat it. She rushed to tell her neighbours who ridiculed and cursed her. Afraid that they would now call her insane as well as barren, she threw the ash into the compost pit.

Twelve years later, Matsyendra Nath decided to visit the child who was his eternal disciple. Visiting the same house, he asked for the boy and was surprised to hear that the woman did not have a child. He asked, "What happened to the ash?" Hearing that the woman had thrown it into the compost pit, he asked to be taken there. He called, "Alakh Niranjan" (one who cannot be seen nor tainted). A young boy emerged from the compost pit and bowing to his master walked away with him.

Gorakh Nath literally means a person who has mastered his *indriyas* or senses and has complete control over the five *vikritis* of human nature - *kaam* (sexuality), *krodh* (temper), *madh* (ego), *lobh* (greed) and *moh* (worldly attachment). Gorakh Nath is regarded as the manifestation of Shiva and is therefore beyond both birth and death. One legend states that Shiva took the form of Gorakh Nath after an argument with Shakti when Shakti told Shiva that she had the power to awaken desire in anyone and Shiva disagreed. In his form as Gorakh Nath, he showed complete freedom from all desires.

Guru Gorakh Nath is thought to have authored the *Goraksha Samhita, Goraksha Sataka, Gorakhsa Sahasra Nama, Gorakhsha Pistika, Goraksha Gita, Amaraugha Prabodha, Jnana Amrita Shastra, Siddha Siddhanta Paddhati, Viveka Martanada, Yoga Martanada, Yoga Siddhanta Paddhati, Yoga-Bija, Yoga Chintamani, Amanaska and Atmabodha,* among other books. He is believed to be the founder of the Nath *Sampradaya* and it is stated that Guru Gorakh Nath has nine Naths and 84 *Siddhas* as disciples, human forms created by his own yogic powers to spread his message of yoga and meditation to the world. He is considered to be ever-existent by Nath Yogis and their followers.

It is widely believed that Guru Gorakh Nath has been alive for thousands of years, watching over the welfare of mankind from behind the scene and occasionally appearing to accomplish a specific goal. In the 19th and 20th centuries, there were several accounts of meetings with him.

When Yogi Sri Shayama Charan Lahiri Mahashaya met "Babaji" in 1861 it is often believed that he met Guru Gorakh Nath. Born in 1828, Lahiri Mahashaya was well-versed in the Vedas and other scriptures and knew several languages, including Sanskrit. At 33, working for the government, he received his transfer orders to report at Ranikhet. One day, enjoying the splendour of the Himalayas, he wandered off the track. Hearing himself addressed familiarly, he met a *yogi* who took him to a cave where Lahiri Mahashaya recalled his previous incarnation as an advanced disciple of his, meditating for decades under his guidance in one of the caves.

The *yogi*, who initiated him into Kriya Yoga, later explained to him that in his present birth he would be instrumental in spreading this knowledge afar. He was assigned the task of setting an example as an ideal *yogi* house-holder, with the responsibility of working and maintaining his family while remaining in spiritual awareness. Lahiri Mahashaya developed many *siddhis* or yogic powers and had numerous disciples, among whom was Sri Yukteshwar Giri, who wrote the *Science of Yoga,* a task assigned to him by Babaji. Later Sri Yukteshwar's disciple, Mahayogi Yogananada was responsible for spreading this message to an international audience.

There are other accounts of meetings with Babaji in many places in Northern India and in the Himalayas between 1861 and 1924. Mahendra Brahmachari spent thirty-five years travelling all over India, collecting stories told about encounters with him. He published these stories titled *"Punya Smriti"* using the pen name Guru Charnasrit. Known by different names in various regions, Babaji was often referred to as Hariakhan Baba. Around 1890, Hariakhan Babaji first appeared publicly. At the time, he was regularly seen by thousands of people and the miraculous events that happened spontaneously around him were witnessed widely. Before and after that, all accounts of him are references of meetings with an individual or a small group.

While details of his appearance varied even when he was observed by several people at the same time, he is generally described as a young man, tall and slender, with light complexion and hair, sometimes worn long and sometimes short. With a noble and dignified appearance, he is described as humble, kind and childlike. He spoke little, was not seen eating anything but *prasad*, and it is said that he never slept. He is described as having unusual physical strength and walked at an extremely rapid pace. His appearances and disappearances were always sudden and unexpected. He conversed readily in different regional languages. He is believed to possess all the known *siddhis* and there are reports of many miracles he performed with natural ease.

There are stories of when he was first seen at Hariakhan village at the foothills of the Himalayas. One night, the people were astonished when they saw a single brilliant light shining from the neighbouring mountain. The mysterious light reappeared on several evenings. Soon the light disappeared from the mountaintop and instead appeared near the village itself. The people gathered to worship the mysterious light and saw a radiant body.

The villagers welcomed him with great respect and it was decided that he would be most comfortable staying with the forest guard, Dham Singh, who lived alone. Singh noticed that the *yogi* would sit still for hours. Not wanting him to be disturbed, he would lock him into the house before leaving for work. One day some of the villagers decided to visit him. They found the house locked. Breaking the lock they went inside but could not find him anywhere. He was not seen again for a decade till he was spotted sitting inside a cave in the depths of the Hariakhan jungle.

Later, he is believed to have lived awhile near the town of Sitlakhet in Almora District. While he was staying there, he asked some disciples where he might find a source of pure cold water. The devotees led him into the forests where there was a trickling spring. He pushed his finger into the earth and water started gushing out. The place where he stayed was named Siddhashram.

A devotee named Siromani Pathak once stayed there overnight. While looking in the direction of the spring he saw what appeared to be four bright flames of light hovering near the stream of water. The whole area was alight from the radiance emanating from the flames, which remained for some time, before disappearing. When Siromani asked Babaji about the lights, he was told that because the place was very sacred, various evolved beings came to the spot and were visible in the form of lights. There are other accounts of people sometimes seeing strange lights in his presence, which they claimed were his saintly visitors.

There are stories about how Maharaja Scindia of Gwalior invited Hariakhan Baba to come to his palace so that he and his wife could have his *darshan.* The king and his ministers met him at the house of a local *pandit* after which he gave *darshan* to the queen at her palace. Interestingly, it is said that the queen had estimated that he was about eighty years old while the king said he had appeared to him to be a mere youth.

There is a story of a time when he was staying near a Shiva temple at Ranibag. In preparation for an auspicious solar eclipse, people had gathered to take a dip in the river Gautami Ganga which ran along the outskirts of the town. They were expecting to take part in a ceremonial bath along with Babaji. Others were keen that he join them for the ritual bath at Kurukshetra, where the famous battle recorded in the Mahabharata had taken place.

Some of the group remained at Ranibag while others went to Kurukshetra. Those at Kurukshetra were delighted to see him wading into the Ganga along with them. When the group returned home to Ranibag, they were surprised to see that he had already arrived back from Kurukshetra. They were told that he had never left.

There are similar accounts in *Autobiography of a Yogi.* There is also an oft-told tale of how Guru Gorakh Nath had found and rescued his *guru* Matsyendra Nath, from Kadali, the land of women. When he returned, he learnt that his *guru* had all along been with some disciples he was teaching. Another legend gives the background to that incident.

The doctrine of *yoga* is said to have been given by Shiva to Baba Gorakh Nath's *guru,* Matsyendra Nath. Legend suggests that Matsyendra Nath, then known as Lokesvara, was thrown into the sea by his parents because he was born on an inauspicious day. Sitting at the seaside, Shiva was teaching the secrets of *yoga* to Parvati. Though Parvati had fallen asleep during the recitation, Lokesvara, who had been swallowed by a fish, heard the entire secret doctrine. Henceforth known as Matsyendra Nath or Lord of the Fish, he was discovered by Shiva who pointed out the eavesdropper to Parvati. She cursed Matsyendra Nath that he would forget all the *yoga* he had learnt in Kadali. Baba Gorakh Nath is supposed to have disguised himself as a dancing girl to rescue Matsyendra Nath from his enchantment.

There are many stories of Babaji told in the Kumaon hills of Uttarakhand, where he is associated with Guru Gorakh Nath, Hariakhan Babaji and other *siddhas*. At the time when he is believed to have stayed at Khurpatal Lake near Nainital, an educated young man speculating on his identity, heard that he had been present at the battle of Kurukshetra which took place over 5,000 years ago. He reasoned that Babaji must really be the immortal warrior, Aswathama. In the Mahabharata it is recorded that Aswathama was wounded on his head. The man figured this must be the reason that he habitually wore a covering on his head.

Excited by his own theory, he sought out Babaji. As soon as Babaji saw the man he suggested a bath in the cool waters of the lake. The young man was delighted at this easy way of ascertaining the truth and looked forward to seeing him remove the cap he wore, when he took his bath. In his presence, however, the man got into a state of trance and as they returned to the hut, he realised he had completely forgotten to look for scars on Babaji's head. The *mahayogi* replied to his unspoken thoughts, "Meet a saint or an evolved soul with respect. Only those blessed by God can recognize a saint. He who has a pure heart attains the grace of saints."

SEEKING OUT THE MASTERS AGAIN

CHAPTER 6

Eternal Quest

"His form is not in the field of vision;
No one sees him with mortal eyes.
He is seen by a pure heart
And by a mind and thoughts that are pure.
Those who know him attain life immortal."

— *Kathopanishad*

Recently while I was talking to a journalist friend of mine, she mentioned that it was *Guru Purnima* the next day. She explained that she regarded 'Babaji' as her *guru.* She could not quite explain who he is. I wrote her the following letter. She replied, "It is the same person."

The Unseen One: He is known as Guru Gorakh Nath. Some call him Mahavtar Babaji, or simply Babaji. He has been referred to as Hariakhan Baba. He is known as the legendary Kripacharya from the days of the Mahabharata.

He stands slender and tall, of an indeterminate age, with a body so subtle that his movements can go unnoticed except by one before whom he chooses to appear. His meditation reverberates in a cosmic sound. His words are few and far between but a single four-word sentence can take lifetimes to unravel.

Mahavtar Babaji is behind the propagation of Kriya Yoga, the renewal of which owes its origin to Mahayogi Yogananda Paramhansa, who received the knowledge of this yogic science from his Guru, Sri Yukteshwar, to whom it had been handed down by Swami Lahiri Mahashaya.

Kriya Yoga was widely practised during the days of the Mahabharata, when *sankalpa shakti* was a known reality. For ages untold, this secret has been guarded in quiet contemplation, until recently, when it has been carried from the recesses of the Himalayas through the whisper of the winds to spread a message of peace.

Kriya Yoga is a rare science and people who practise it are few and far between. They enjoy the special protection of the sages of the Himalayas. The initial practice of Kriya Yoga has been made available for the uninitiated, but care has to be taken to learn from one who knows the discipline. The ultimate secrets of this science are revealed only to the very few who are ready for the teaching.

Guru Gorakh Nath has been a guiding spirit in my life. Both Pilot Baba and Gorakh Baba have given me the vision of eternity that I have always known, often unconsciously. With others, too, have I shared an eternal space, beyond the bondage of time and space, of birth and death. To take embodiment in the Realm of Mankind, to live in the Paradise of Innocence, to Manifest the Creations of the Mind in Awareness and to seek the Unmanifest—this then is my Eternal Quest.

CHAPTER 7

Crisis of Faith

"He cannot be seen by the eye,
And words cannot reveal him.
He cannot be reached by the senses,
Or by austerity or sacred actions.
By the grace of wisdom and purity of mind,
He can be seen indivisible in the silence of contemplation."

— *Mundaka Upanishad*

Twelve years after I had last met Pilot Baba, I wrote a letter to him:

"Dear Pilot Baba,

A long time ago I had written about my meetings with you. I have recently written something about Mahavtar Babaji, which I have not yet published and am sending to you. Unsure of the direction of the work before me, I need your guidance, directions and blessings, and that of Babaji.

I would like to meet you again to understand anew the secrets of eternity, which I believe I have earnestly sought with my life, armed with Babaji's words to me, "Life is a question. Solve it."

My deepest regards,
Romola"

Pilot Baba was abroad at the time I wrote to him. I followed his movements over several months through his devoted disciple, Hariom. When he returned to India, I was still not able to meet him, though I did speak to him on the phone once, when he assured me that we would meet soon. At intervals, Hariom would write to me. He sent me a mail:

"Hi Romola,

Greetings.

I talked to Babaji who gave a message for you to continue your meditation and that he will meet you after returning from the Himalayas. Babaji sends his blessings to you. He will meet you when the time comes.

Bye

Hariom"

In my reply to Hariom, I wrote:

"Please tell Pilot Babaji that I have only ever meditated with my life, so as long as I am living I hope I am meditating. I would be grateful if you could also convey my humble thanks to him for his blessings.

"May his blessings be with me that I have the courage, patience and determination to live in different realms without understanding and to live in the void without wisdom, until my time comes. May his blessings be with me that I may recognise the Divine, again and again, and be able to endure the pain of separation without forgetfulness until the next time of recognition, that I have the humility to surrender to the will of the Divine, have the discrimination to know the relative from the absolute, that I may understand the meaning of life and fulfil the purpose of my life. And above all, for Grace."

In the meantime, my own spiritual journey had taken me back to Almora to meet my old friend, Mashima, affectionately called Mataji by everyone there. She had often regaled me with tales of her life experiences and shared her spiritual insights, at the time that I was absorbed in the study of philosophy and scriptural texts while seeking an experiential learning through life itself.

During my visit, I revealed to her that I was keen to learn Kriya Yoga. She warned me that Kriya Yoga must be learnt from one who knows the discipline. She mentioned that her *guru* was an adept but that she herself had never been curious about it. She also told me that the Maharaj at Mukhteshwar, whom I had met several years earlier, also practised Kriya Yoga, but that he was presently in Kolkata. She said that Kriya Yoga could be learnt only with a steadfast mind. It was walking the razor's edge, with death and insanity as the precipice on either side.

One day, sitting talking to her, I fell asleep and when I awoke she said, "I saw a tired child. I think we both needed this meeting." In parting she said, "Even the wrong path takes you to the same destination, if followed with sincerity. Let me give you the same blessings given to me by the Mukhteshwar Maharaj, when I visited him last, during a period of doubt. You are on the path. The path itself will reveal the way ahead. May the meaning of life unfold and blossom before you."

I went to Mukteshwar on my way back from Almora. I could hardly recognise the simple temple and the *gufa* where the Maharaj used to live. The place had developed considerably. In the local buses, I noticed pictures of him. It was no wonder the Maharaj had shifted base to Kolkata.

I recall when we met him several years ago. We had been forewarned that he rarely met anyone. He would emerge from his cave to give brief *darshan* at sunset. It was a chilly winter evening and the clouds hemmed in. We waited. The *yogi*, dressed in white cotton *dhoti-kurta*, with a flowing grey beard, was observing *mauna* for several years. He raised his hand in blessing as a handful of waiting people went one by one to him. A waiting *sadhu*, also obviously observing silence, wrote on a slate, and the Maharaj replied on the same slate. It was our turn. I requested permission to talk to him. He looked at me intently and indicated that he would call us soon.

He invited us into his cave. After he replied to a few questions by writing on a slate, he suddenly asked me whether my enquiries were mere curiosity or whether I was sincere in my search. Obviously satisfied with my reply, he indicated that the weather had turned foul and that we should take young Siddhartha back, before it grew too dark. On his slate he wrote that if we could stay another day, he would meet us the following day. I requested permission to bring paper and pen, since the slate was a slow process. Erudite and well versed in the scriptures, he had an easy style of writing and was equally fluent in English, Hindi and Bengali.

The next day we were invited into his cave and given hot cups of tea before we settled down to a philosophical discussion conducted in writing. After a couple of hours of reading and writing by the glow of the lamp, I heard a rasping hoarse voice, barely audible from years of not using his vocal chords. I looked at him in surprise, and reminded him of his *mauna*. He smiled and dismissed it as unimportant, that he would be able to convey what he had to say better this way. I acknowledged his blessing.

Years later, standing at the same place, I watched the setting sun and smiled at the little notice outside his *kutia*, which requested the observance of silence. And the silence spoke.

Returning to Mumbai, it seemed to me that I was compelled to seek the meaning of life without a glimmer of hope on the horizon. I was spontaneously drawn towards Kriya Yoga. I could not reconcile the different facets of living and I felt quite fragile. In the world around me, surrounded by worldly values and goals, it seemed to me that the inner voice that had always guided me had fallen ominously silent. My husband, Rajiv and a close friend, both separately expressed concern when they said the same words, "I see a lost child."

I found myself surrounded by other people's losses, anxieties, miseries, conflicts and grief. In my confusion I seemed to have lost my own ability to offer solace. In a conversation with a friend, I expressed my reservations, stating that I was in the lowest phase of my life.

He asked, "What has placed you at this level?"

"Life, I guess and the fact that I was surprised by it. I am being forced to see different perspectives. At this point none seem pleasurable and I do not know how to garner the energy to seek answers. But I would rather do it now than have to return again!" I said. "I am compelled to live without anchors, or at least to realise the transience of everything in life. I have lost the one anchor I always had...a sense of God. What can you ask for from the Unmanifest?" I enquired.

"The glory that life offers, what else?" said my friend. "To be alone, while in harmony with the whole at the same time. To share the grace, wisdom and energy you have known. You have seen the wonders that life offers. The mould you come from does not allow stagnation or a state of limbo, a sheltered state. You seek growth and joy, therefore, you must also experience the opposite, as neither stands alone. You will not appreciate light without knowing the dark."

CHAPTER 8

Bharatpur Calls

"The real voyage of discovery consists not in seeking new landscapes but in having new eyes."

—*Marcel Proust*

Old and in frail health, my parents desperately wanted me to visit Kolkata as soon as possible. My brother and sister-in-law had come from the U.S. for a holiday. I had planned that I would visit them in Kolkata, after which I intended to head towards the Garhwal hills of Uttarakhand.

I needed time off from city living and stresses. I wanted to get in touch again with an inner core of spirituality, because for the first time in my life, I was feeling a deep crisis of faith. Till recently, I had never experienced any conflict in taking decisions. I always knew what I had to do next. I do not remember having wondered which of two choices I should take: the choice was always inevitable and obvious, guided by the hands of a destiny that I was comfortable to surrender to.

On the day of my scheduled departure, in the midst of packing and trying to organise the house to run with some degree of efficiency in my absence, Rajiv, who was checking my e-mail for me, said, "There is a mail from Hari Om. Do you want to read it?" I came and stood beside him as we read the mail together. It said:

"Hi Romola,

Greetings.

Babaji has a *yagna* programme in Bharatpur, near Mathura, from 17th to 25th October. He said that

I should write to you telling you that you are cordially invited to the programme. There is also a *samadhi* programme from 20th to 24th. Try to come if possible as you know how difficult it is to trace Babaji.

Greetings again.

Regards,

Hari"

Did I have an alternative but to go? I checked online for trains to Mathura, and we hurriedly left for the station, almost sure that tickets would not be available. Standing in a queue, I secured waitlisted tickets, and then stood in another queue to cancel my Kolkata tickets. Rajiv wandered off to check the availability of onward reservations for Kolkata. He returned to say that a flash on a screen said that seventy tickets had been released on the August Kranti. My ticket to Mathura was confirmed.

I rang up and told my mother I would be arriving in Kolkata 10 days later, without offering an explanation for why my trip was delayed. I had spoken to her the previous night confirming that I was reaching my childhood home. I knew she would be extremely disappointed.

The brief time before the train left, I felt strangely relieved, sure I was doing the right thing. I could look at the traffic in Mumbai again, without feeling that growing sense of congestion and suffocation. I watched people hurrying along with their lives without seeing misery written large on their faces. I was ready to embrace life again.

At Mathura, where the train stopped briefly, I disembarked and took a rickshaw to the bus station from where buses to Bharatpur plied regularly. I had been told by Hari Om, whom I called in Delhi, that the *yagna* would be at Mohan Mandir, Quila, Bharatpur. He added that if I went there it would not be difficult to make staying arrangements. He mentioned that Pilot Baba would be in Bharatpur the day after I arrived.

At the ticket counter, on enquiry, I was told which bus to take to my destination, and introduced to the conductor who promised to tell me where to get off. I had visited the Bird Sanctuary many years ago. I travel easily and lightly, soaking in the atmosphere of different places. I was relaxed and enjoyed the drive, oblivious of the crowded bus. The tree-lined roads with long stalks of heather rippling in the breeze fanned my sense of familiarity with this and other roads I have travelled. At a crossing at Bharatpur the bus turned, and the conductor suggested that I take a rickshaw for the *Quila,* or Fort, which I did.

At the mandir, I found the priest sitting in the ample courtyard within the temple precinct, with several people surrounding him. I am not at all familiar with temples, preferring to offer worship through a spontaneous appreciation of nature, through expressions of joy. There was an air of neglect and a sense of controlled oppression. Later I learnt that exorcism was practised here.

On enquiry, it was suggested that I go across the road to find out about the *yagna.* Leaving my travelling bag at the *mandir,* I went across to the advocate's house opposite and enquired if Pilot Baba was there. I was given no information and instead told, "The Raja Saheb is inside. You cannot go in." Requesting that a message be given to Pilot Baba that I had arrived from Mumbai, I stood a few seconds before being ushered in. I quickly spotted Pilot Baba, whom I had not met for more than twelve years. I did *pranam* to him for the first time ever. I am not readily given to doing *pranam.* For me it is a gesture of the highest respect offered with total sincerity.

Sitting down, I was introduced as a journalist from Mumbai. I was offered coffee, which I gladly accepted. I sank into my chair to view the proceedings. It was a motley crowd from widely divergent backgrounds, most of whom sat in attentive discomfort. Vishvendra Singh, heir of the erstwhile Maharajas of Bharatpur and a twice elected M.P., made polished drawing room conversation that I could easily relate to. Pilot Baba, always relaxed, yet alert, dominated the room with his presence. He pointed towards plates of *mithai* and *dalmoth*, which I declined. Ram Narayan Das, at whose instance the *yagna* was being held at Bharatpur, chided me, "You do not refuse what Babaji offers. It is *prasad*." I had unintentionally made a gaffe.

Babaji quickly defended me with characteristic generosity of spirit, "It is okay. She is Bhagwati Ma and has been to Pindari." I took a little piece of the proffered sweetmeat that had been the focus of this conversation. After this, despite my unconventional dress code in jeans, shirt and walking shoes, and despite my obvious language barrier in the heartland of the Hindi belt, more familiar as I am with English than Hindi, and despite all the prerequisites of acceptability that were lacking, I was treated as a member of Babaji's '*parivar*' or family.

I soon met all the people accompanying him with whom I had ample opportunity to interact at leisure, over several days. Among the women, there was Kusum, sensitive and reserved, who accepted me as a confidante. I spent many hours with her, one way or another, discussing her life and circumstances; attempting to unravel the psyche of one who has dedicated herself to becoming a *sanyasini*; trying to understand the intricacies of life in an *ashram*; sharing knowledge and wisdom in whatever form it presented itself.

Chetna had a rare poise and supreme self-confidence. At 23, she had already taken public *samadhi* three times. She told me her life story with guileless honesty, talked of her experiences of *samadhi* with disarming candour, invited me to be present at her next *samadhi* and hugged me with warmth and without reservation, when I finally left.

I spent the least amount of time with calm and serene Chandra, mentally absorbed as she was in preparing for her first public *samadhi*. She isolated herself days before going underground into the pit. She remained in *samadhi* for a predetermined seventy two hours, before she emerged rested and tranquil. I noticed no visible difference in her. I saw in her the innocence of childhood and the faith of one who can surrender her very life in belief.

Subsequently, I got to know all three of them better and spent wonderful times with them. I also got to know some of the others. Mangal Giri Maharaj looks after Baba's ashram at the foothills of Nainital. I had the opportunity of spending time with him at Pipariya before he took *samadhi* there. Calm, quiet and unassuming, he is observant and expresses himself with frank honesty.

Swami Avdeshananda, initially preoccupied with his introspections, is an interesting conversationalist with a keen intellect. I found him to be thoughtful, self-assured and determined. Nilu Maharaj is practical, hard-working and energetic while being devoted to his spiritual pursuits. A householder, he accompanies Baba for *yagnas* and is an efficient organiser. Extremely pleasant and helpful, he has an easy manner and laughs readily. Kamtaji, an elderly devotee of Baba who is a social worker and has been an MLA, also accompanies Baba for *yagnas.* Protective about Baba's welfare, he keeps his own counsel and takes his time to be friendly. He is a keen observer with a determined and detached sense of purpose. Sharmaji has spent close to two decades with Babaji and drives his vehicle on his travels. He is outspoken and aloof, an insider who is a perpetual outsider.

BLESSINGS OF THE MASTERS

CHAPTER 9

Guru Gorakh Nath's Blessings

"He comes to the thought of those
Who know him beyond thought,
Not to those who imagine he can be attained by thought."

— *Kena Upanishad*

The afternoon of my arrival, in a gesture of welcome, I was rewarded with the uninterrupted attention of Pilot Baba as I sat for several hours in his room, talking, listening, seeking guidance, assimilating knowledge and absorbing wisdom. He asked me, "Why have you not written?" I replied, "Because..." and as I marshalled my thoughts in explanation, he said, "Because you have not realised?" As I nodded and said I needed to have my writing confirmed before I could share it, he said, "Write our conversations."

That perhaps is where this tale begins. Or perhaps it began ages ago, in remembrances of *samadhis* known.

We talked of Gorakh Baba. I repeated what I had rarely shared. That I had lived twelve years with his single advice, "Life is a question. Solve it." Once in the midst of living, I had thought, "I can no longer seek this truth. I will postpone it for another lifetime". I remembered well that Pilot Baba had remarked about my state of awareness that evening years ago at Khati, in the presence of Gorakh Baba, "When you leave this body, if it is with this awareness, you will not take birth again." I had affirmed that I believed that. Not in arrogance, but in humility at the blessing given. I understood clearly that I had been warned, as well as promised, that there was much living ahead that would have to be undertaken with understanding.

Yet, I was giving up the search in this lifetime, because my *karmas* seemingly held me bound. I have lived my life offering my *karmas* in the flame of knowledge, which alone purifies us to go beyond. Yet it seemed to me that I was fulfilling *karmic* impressions so compelling that they held me in their sway. I prayed with sincerity.

Picking up a book, I opened it and found an admonishment that we must not postpone accomplishing our goal until the next lifetime. It was written that Guru Gorakh Nath emphatically states, "Shame on the aspirant who claims to be sincere but dies before accomplishing the purpose of his life. And shame on the teacher who says he is a *sadguru* (adept) and who allows his disciple to die before he accomplishes the purpose of his life."

I had immediately thought, Pilot Baba had said that I would not have a *guru.* I had long believed that God is my *guru.* Did I doubt that God had the ability to cross me to the other shore through the sea of *samsara*? I could not give up and live in forgetfulness. I was prepared to seek spiritual answers in the mire of daily living.

I had lost the Self I had always held dear, because of whom all else appears dear. I had lost the God I could pray to since my earliest memories of childhood prayer. That was a personal God, a friend, familiar, who knew me well, whom I could trust to point the way.

Within myself I had lost the ability to discriminate between Truth and Untruth, between the path that leads to Ignorance and the one that leads to Knowledge, between the path that leads to Darkness in a world of Illusion and that which leads to an everlasting Light. But I still sought answers of Death that would lead me to Immortality, while I spun between the *karmic* cycles of living.

Now, a world away, I was talking again of Gorakh Baba to one who knew him well. When Gorakh Baba walked into the room, almost without greeting, it was as though he had just walked out the door and was re-entering it now. As he quietly sat down near Pilot Baba, I bent and touched the ground before his feet in homage, as I had done when I met Pilot Baba.

Pilot Baba asked him, "*Bitia ko pehchana*?" (Do you recognise her?).

I introduced myself by saying that I had meditated with my life for twelve years with his words to me, "Life is a question".

Pilot Baba started to translate my words in Hindi, as I recalled he had done at our earlier meeting when I had first spoken to Gorakh Baba. He looked at me closely before he laughed spontaneously. I saw again for a few brief moments the person who had spoken twelve years ago. "Life is also the answer," he said in English, as he had done earlier.

"I know that," I said too quickly, probably reluctant to let another twelve years lapse before the next lesson were given!

"You will find all the answers," he assured me in benediction.

That was all I needed to know from Gorakh Baba. However, the next day, Gorakh Baba taught me much more in silence, with his actions and his behaviour. His words touched the very core of my being. His touch upon my head when I bowed before him in reverence was not merely a blessing. It was also a promise.

Chapter 10

A Master is a Bridge

**"As rivers flowing into the ocean find their final peace
And their name and form disappear,
Even so the wise become free from name and form
And enter into the radiance of the Supreme Spirit
Who is greater than all greatness."**

—*Mundaka Upanishad*

In the afternoon I sat before Pilot Baba, my empty hands offered in a gesture of supplication to a master. I said, "I come to you with empty hands." I was aware that I had come to him as a student seeking Knowledge and Wisdom.

He said, "That is good. Then there is space to fill them. If they are already full, they will overflow."

I reminded him that he had told me years ago that I would not have a *guru*. "Without a *guru* it is difficult indeed to tread this path," I said.

"A master is only a bridge to help you cross," he replied simply.

Pilot Baba spoke of the Ultimate Truth of the Upanishads. "You are not the body and you are not the mind. You are the Self beyond both." He went on to explain, "Be a witness and you will separate yourself from both. This is the body and you can watch it. That is the mind and it is conditioned by society. Every thought involves someone else or what has been taught to you by someone else."

I lamented that the world today is caught in an ever-growing trap of materialism. Almost petulantly, I said, "I don't want to touch money."

Amused, he teased, "Why? It is not the Self who deals with money." But then he blessed me, "Money will never affect you. As it cannot affect me. We already know its colour."

As if I knew a secret of some great importance, which he may not know, I said, "There are people who live in the world, who have forgotten who they are."

With seeming callousness, he said, "Let them suffer. It is their own *karma.*" At the same time, he reminded me, "You will not suffer if you are enlightened. As a witness, you will enjoy everything." Seeing my inability to reconcile the path of individual salvation from the human condition of suffering, he relented, "If you love someone, you can remind them to recognise themselves. Challenge them, cause them pain. Suffering brings it's own freedom."

I asked him, "Can anyone change the course of a river?"

He replied, "Yes, if you love someone, you can."

Almost as though he spoke to himself, he said, "Before the river merges into the ocean, it becomes very wide."

He said, "No one else can make you recognise yourself. Dive deep within yourself and you will be enlightened."

Recalling the last time he had told me to dive, I told him how I had overcome my extreme and acute fear of water and gone scuba diving. The first time I dived, my mind had opened to a new ecstasy. It was so incredibly beautiful. I knew why I was there. I am the Ocean, I had said. I am. I know. And so I dived into the ocean to find another realm. An eternity that cannot be logged in minutes. Another space beyond dimensions. In speechless wonder, I saw beauty and perfection. I crossed the threshold of my fears to know a new freedom.

Pilot Baba said, "Now dive within yourself. Remember that you are not the body and you are not the mind. Be a witness. Go into the darkness. If you seek the gods, you will only find the gods. Expect nothing. And you will recognise yourself. But go without even asking who you are. Meditate and go into that total darkness."

I wanted to know, "But having gone, how do I return?"

He smiled at my fears, as though to ask, "Does it matter?" I understood immediately why he had smiled. How could I possibly go into that Darkness, leaving everything behind, if I was already looking for the exit lights?

His next words reminded me of the Knowledge I was unconsciously seeking, "You only return from love. As the Buddha did. And Christ. And Mahavir...." he said, naming a few of the known enlightened masters.

"Your heart is open. You have no attachments. You are ready," he said, reminding me that I had dropped everything and heeded the imperative call.

I admitted, "I still have some attachments." I particularly mentioned a conversation I once had with my son, Siddhartha, when I had asked him if I had his permission to live in seclusion if my search so demanded. I had said to him, "I will not go, if you want me to stay."

The wisdom of his reply had startled me, "Mama, even if I told you not to go, you should not stop for that."

Listening to a recounting of the incident, Pilot Baba now said, "What a beautiful way to set you free."

Recognising that I still felt trapped by karmic impressions whose fetters I was not released from, he explained, "Apart from our own karmic attachments, there are attachments generated by the karmic impressions of those whose lives are entangled with ours."

To help me unravel the knots of my karmic impressions, he gave me a treasured knowledge that I had sought hard, though I had not mentioned it to him. He said, "I will teach you some kriyas that will help you on the path to enlightenment. When it will happen, I cannot say. That depends on your own readiness. On how open your heart is."

"Enlightenment comes at once, not in flashes," he said from the depths of his being, explaining to me almost instantaneously the difference between glimpses of truth and enlightenment. I now understood that glimpses of truth compel us to seek the path towards enlightenment. Baba said, "No one else can give you realisation."

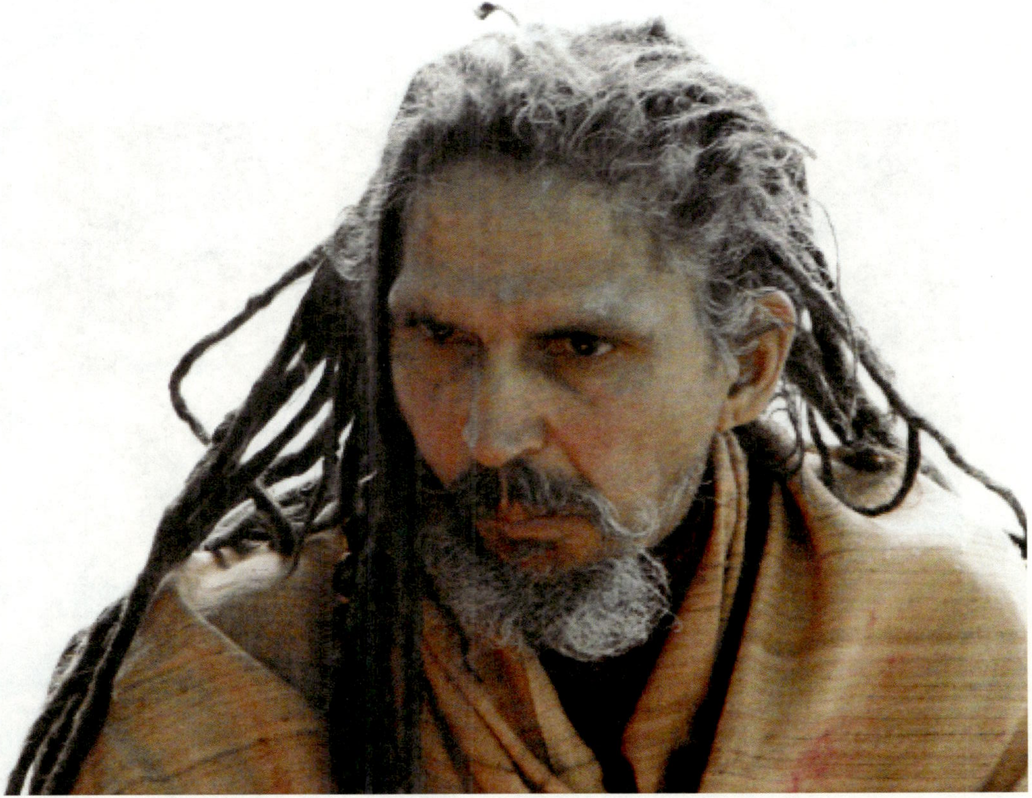

GORAKH BABAJI

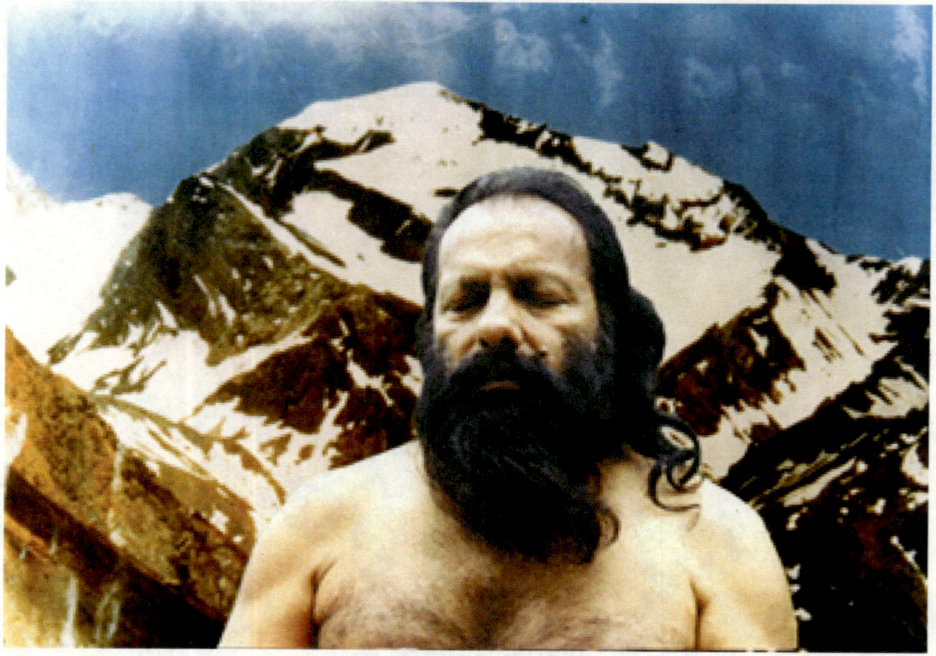

PILOT BABAJI - AT AUM PARBAT

In the presence of Gorakh Baba, who sat mostly in silence, I looked at the contemporary clothes I am comfortable wearing, and at the saffron cloths draped on Pilot Baba, "I would not wear anything else," I said, stating my own reservations and misgivings of having to conform to any expectations.

Very gently Pilot Baba said, "True *sanyas* is total freedom." And then he spoke of saffron as the symbol of fire, and I understood that it is a reminder of the fires they have crossed.

As evening started to fall, we went out and sat on the lawn. We were soon joined by several *sadhus*, many of whom sat talking to Pilot Baba, seeking clarification for their doubts. Gorakh Baba watched in silence, before leaving quite suddenly without a word, but having clearly indicated his departure.

Chapter 11

Glimpses of Truth

From joy all beings have come,
By joy they all live,
And unto joy they return."

— *Taittiriya Upanishad*

In retrospect, I remember many shared truths with seekers I have met in Life. They crossed my path on different walks of life. They always stopped to share their wisdom. Their blessings have been bountiful.

The only blessing I have consciously sought is that I may know, understand and recognise. On the way I have received many more. Some were boons of protection against the pitfalls of living in a world of Ignorance.

More than twenty years ago, an ascetic came to the door of our house in Kanpur, and said, "Do not deny God in any form that he comes to you. God sent me to you."

Rajiv had replied, "If I recognise him, I will surely not deny him."

To which the ascetic replied, "Recognise him" and offered a boon, "Ask me for anything you want."

Rajiv said to him, "*Yeh safar kat jai.*" (May this journey be completed).

He replied, "*Aap sant ho.*" (You are a saint). He continued, "May you be protected against all evil. May your enemies be destroyed."

Rajiv said, "Let them also live."

He repeated, "*Aap sant ho.*" Then modified his boon, "May evil be destroyed when it comes within reach of you."

Does a greater boon exist in the world of living?

He blessed us, "You will never know the need for food, for clothes, for money." I hoped not for a surfeit of worldly possessions, but that I would never be aware of their absence. I have always received in greater plenty than my needs.

Several times when we watched the sunset at Bright End Corner in Almora, we would notice a bricklayer absorbed in reverie as the sun sank behind the mountains, leaving an orange glow. A few months later, on our way to Binsar, we met him beside his shelter. He was now wearing saffron.

Dusk had fallen and we had to walk the remaining 3 km distance to where we had been invited for the weekend. At the time, Siddhartha, was a three-year-old fearless child of the Himalayas. The mendicant stopped us, lit a fire and gave us excellent hot tea before insisting that he guide us through the deep, dense forests, shared by panthers, in the dark and cold of that winter night. He clutched the *trishul* he carried with him and visibly sought to conquer his fears with a chanting of *mantras.* Months later, meeting him briefly again near the marketplace at Almora, he stopped to say, "We return because of love."

Years ago, in the midst of transferring residence from one city to another, we travelled in our overloaded car and stopped at a makeshift tyre shop on the way, to change a puncture. The tall, strong, elderly man in long grey hair and beard, who repaired it, was clad as a renunciate. As he collected his dues he enquired, "Where do you come from?"

Rajiv said, "Bareilly. I am on my way to Lucknow."

The man laughed spontaneously and said, "I have more experience than that." He explained, "I was asking you where you belong." He smiled and waved us on with blessings, while asking, "Do you remember who you are?"

Several years ago, friends from New Zealand were visiting and wanted to donate a small sum of money to Mother Theresa's Sisters of Charity. I had taken them to 'Mother Home' and stated the purpose of our visit. We waited. Mother

Theresa arrived and greeted us. Her bowed shoulders and weather-beaten face spoke of years in the service of Jesus. She folded her hands together in acceptance of the offering with a humility I have rarely seen in anyone. She said, "Visit the orphanage. Contact with the poor is good."

Anyone who has visited Mother Theresa's homes, be it for children or for the destitute, knows that it is always an intensely humbling experience. To dedicate oneself to the service of mankind and serve the poorest of the poor must open the gates of heaven.

Visiting Mirtola Ashram during the time when Sri Madhav Ashish was looking after the *ashram*, we spent an afternoon in the quiet serene atmosphere there. Before leaving, Sri Madhav Ashish gave me a copy of *Yoga of the Kathopanishad*, written by his *guru* Sri Krishna Prem, mentioning that it was out of print.

The *Kathopanishad* has long been one of my favourite Upanishads. It is one I have sought to understand at every turn of the way, aware that some of the mysteries of the universe can be understood by standing at Yama's door, as Nachiketa did. Or by meditating on the fearsome ascetic, Shiva and demanding, "I have come to you to learn the secrets of Immortality, which you have guarded so well."

KRIYA YOGA

CHAPTER 12

Initiation into Kriya Yoga

**"This calm steadiness of the senses is called Yoga.
Then one should become watchful,
Because Yoga comes and goes"**

— *Kathopanishad*

Pilot Baba asked me to meet him before 6 in the morning so he could teach me a few *kriyas.* When I reached where he was staying, in the glimmer of first light, he was walking barefoot on the grass. While a new dawn broke, he taught me what I needed to know, saying, "These are very powerful. Anything can happen when you practise them. Anything."

He taught me the invocations in English. They had obviously been modified to suit my individual needs, so when I struggled to remember his words the next day, I realised that the form was less important than the natural flow of prayers that sprang from my heart. The prayers were very simple. They were the expression of oft-repeated silent prayers that had always been a part of my own nature.

He taught me two different versions of a particular *kriya,* which I practised before him. He explained that I should choose one or the other at any time while practising it. "This is a powerful *kriya,*" he explained. He added that I could practise it along with the repetition of the *mantra,* "*Aum*", if I so wished.

After that he taught me *kriya pranayama,* which are a series of breathing exercises that lead to awareness and control of the life force. He explained that these would enable fitness of heart, lungs and head, while promoting awareness.

The next *kriya* I learnt would facilitate the knowledge I had sought a long time. Pilot Baba said, "this will take you beyond death." It involved the arousing of the *Kundalini.* He explained how to allow awareness to arise to the highest point of consciousness in the head.

After that he gave me guidance on my meditation practice. He knew my sincerity. He was also aware of my free-spiritedness. He always asked me questions. I spoke without hesitation about what I believe. Accordingly, he taught me the *kriyas* in the manner that would be most beneficial for me.

I would faithfully follow my *kriya* practices in the time to come. And live in the world without any restrictions whatsoever. I found myself stepping back into the familiar practice of meditating with my life. I was now aware that I should be a witness to the fullest extent that I could.

I bowed before him, deeply aware of what he had shared with me. My silent prayers are that I may never forget the purpose for which I sought this knowledge, that of recognising the Self to be enlightened. My sincere prayers are that I may always be aware of my body, my mind, my senses and my consciousness so that caught in illusory mayic cycles, I never misuse the powers that the *kriyas* generate.

CHAPTER 13

An Ancient Esoteric Science

"When in the Yoga of holy contemplation
The movements of the mind and the breath of life
Are in a harmony of peace,
There is steadiness,
And that steadiness is pure."

— *Bhagavad Gita*

The Himalayas have protected practitioners of the ancient science of Kriya Yoga. Knowledge of this esoteric science has been kept safe and intact with the great Himalayan saints who understand this technique and who impart this knowledge, according to the needs of the time, through the medium of chosen *yogis*. Various feats like taking *samadhi* for centuries, sudden appearance and disappearance and the creation of multiple bodies are possible only through Kriya Yoga.

The Sanskrit word *kriya* means "action." In Patanjali's two thousand year old treatise on the Yoga Sutras, *Kriya Yoga* is defined as the disciplined regulation of mental and sensory impulses, self-analysis, study of metaphysics, meditation, and surrender of self-consciousness in favor of cosmic consciousness.

Kriya Yoga is a complete system covering a wide range of techniques, including prayer, mantras, meditation, pranayama and awakening of the *Kundalini*. Geared towards control of life force, this science enables a human being to have control over his thought processes. It consists of systematic, well-defined techniques to promote spiritual enlightenment. Kriya Yoga practice generates awareness of wholeness through knowledge of one's spiritual nature, promotes rational thinking, emotional balance and physical health. To facilitate the awakening of super-conscious states, specific meditation techniques are taught and practised. The goal is to unite with pure Awareness, our original condition.

Kriya Yoga is a secret science divulged by the *rishis* and *munis* after proof of one's worthiness to be taught the nuances of this intricate science. It involves the science of laya and *vilaya* or harmony and disintegration of thoughts. It creates the necessary framework for cognition of s*ankalpit yoga.* Through the mastery of *sankalpit yoga,* man can lead a life of free will. Even the slightest misuse of the power can be extremely disastrous and history has shown that its misuse leads to destruction.

According to Puranic history, Lord Shiva first taught Kriya Yoga to Parvati. Lord Rama learnt Kriya Yoga from Guru Vashista. Shiva is believed to have initiated both Ravana and Markandey into *kriya.* Ravana misused the powers of this great science and was consequently destroyed.

Lord Krishna was an adept of Kriya Yoga. All his mayic activities illustrate his mastery of these techniques. Through Kriya Yoga a man can obtain the state of *sankalpi*t *yoga,* an extremely powerful weapon. The colossal misuse of *sankalpit yoga* caused havoc in the times of the Mahabharata when *Kriya Yoga* had become accessible to common people who had thereby acquired miraculous powers.

Explaining the lineage through which Kriya Yoga techniques were passed on, Pilot Baba says, "Bhagwan Bhaśkar gave *kriya diksha* to Vivaswan, the Sun, who revealed it to his son, Manu, the father of Man. Manu handed it over to his son, King Ikshvaku. Shardwan received the knowledge from him. It remained in oblivion till Parshuram revived it. Dronacharya received it from Parshuram. Ashwathma learnt the rare art from Dronacharya. Bhishma Pitamah and others who played a significant role in the events of the Mahabharata, were also versed in Kriya Yoga. Kripacharya and Kripi, later known as Shanti Ma, received it from Shardwan."

Mahayogi Kapil Advait says, "After the Mahabharata, Kriya Yoga went into hibernation and has been reawakened after a lapse of five thousand years. We owe the revival of Kriya Yoga to Mahayogi Yoganandaji, who was initiated by his *guru*, Sri Yukteshwar who learnt it from Swami Lahiri Mahashaya who was taught by Mahavtar Baba, who is the legendary Kripacharya."

Pilot Baba says, "Today, man wants to embrace everything without delay, overlooking the fact that nothing can be achieved in a hurry. Kriya Yoga has many practical aspects that can contribute to the development of human consciousness. It's chief objective is to instil love for mankind. It intends to purify the practitioner's thoughts so he can be a source of inspiration for others. *Sankalpit yoga* can change the course of probable events that can destroy mankind. The great sages have decided to curtail the use of destructive power that threatens society today. The Himalayas remain quiet and unperturbed. Man can attempt anything. Finally, it is the will of God that will prevail."

CHAPTER 14

Practice of Kriya Yoga

The word is *Aum*
Reflection upon its meaning reveals the Way
From this comes the realisation of the Self.

—*Yoga Sutras of Patanjali*

Explaining a few basic precepts of Kriya Yoga, Pilot Baba says, "The practice of Kriya Yoga is very effective in breaking our ties with the external world. When a practitioner gets absorbed in his divinity, he begins to experience divine sparks. This world bathed in yellow light is the gift of spiritual attainments. When the *sadhak* enters into this world, he comes very close to the ultimate goal.

"He attains mastery over his will through the continual practice of this technique. Subsequently, he achieves excellence in controlling his thoughts. Thus, he obtains the stage of *sankalpit yoga.* With the power of his thought vibrations he can change the impossible into possible. He can arrest the race of his thoughts as well as control all bodily functions and enter into *samadhi.* He achieves free will and can easily enter and exit the gross body."

The science of Kriya Yoga became widely known in modern India through the instrumentality of Lahiri Mahashaya. The Sanskrit root of *kriya* is *kri,* to do, to act and react; the same root is found in the word *karma,* the natural principle of cause and effect. Kriya Yoga is the union (*yoga*) with the Infinite through a certain action or rite, termed *kriya.* A *yogi* who faithfully practices the technique is gradually freed from *karma* or the chain that causes equilibrium through the laws of cause and effect.

Kriya Yoga is a simple, psycho-physiological method by which human blood is decarbonised and recharged with oxygen. The atoms of this extra oxygen are transmuted into life current to rejuvenate the brain and spinal centres. By stopping the accumulation of venous blood, the *yogi* is able to lessen or prevent the decay of tissues and transmute his cells into energy.

Kriya Yoga is mentioned by the ancient sage and exponent of yoga, Patanjali who wrote: "Kriya Yoga consists of body discipline, mental control and meditating on *Aum.*" Patanjali speaks of God as the actual cosmic sound of *Aum* that is heard in meditation. *Aum* is the primordial sound, the creative word and the perpetual witness of divine presence.

In the initial states, the practitioner's consciousness merges with the cosmic spirit; his life force is withdrawn from the body, which remains motionless and rigid. The *yogi* is fully aware of his bodily condition of suspended animation. As he progresses to higher spiritual states, he can commune with God in his ordinary waking consciousness.

The scriptures say that man requires a million years of normal evolution to perfect his human brain sufficiently to express cosmic consciousness. The ancient *rishis* discovered that there are twelve-year cycles that impel one towards the spiritual unfolding of knowledge.

Statistically, it has been stated that one thousand *kriyas* practiced in about eight hours gives the *yogi*, in one day, the equivalent of one thousand years of natural evolution. It has been estimated that in three years an advanced *kriya yogi*, well versed in the practice, can accomplish what nature brings to pass in a million years. With proper guidance, a *yogi* can systematically prepare his body and brain to withstand the power generated by intensive practice.

The rejuvenating effects of sleep are due to man's temporary unawareness of body and breathing. During sleep, one's breath flows more slowly and evenly. The sleeping man becomes a *yogi*; each night he unconsciously performs the *yogic* rite of releasing himself from bodily identification and of merging the life force with healing currents in the main brain region and in the six sub-dynamos of his spinal centres. Unknowingly, the sleeper is thus recharged by the cosmic energy that sustains all life.

The *yogi* performs a simple, natural process consciously. A *kriya yogi* uses this technique to saturate and feed all his physical cells with light energy and thus keeps them in a spiritually magnetised state. He scientifically makes breathing unnecessary and does not enter the negative states of sleep, unconsciousness, or death, during his hours of practice.

Untying the cord of breath that binds the soul to the body, *kriya* serves to prolong life and to enlarge individual consciousness to unite with cosmic consciousness. Yoga helps overcome the constant attraction between mind and matter and senses. The *yogi* can experience himself without nature's elemental compulsions. Master of his body and mind, the *kriya yogi* ultimately overcomes death, achieving recognition of his own immortality.

UNDERSTANDING THE KATHOPANISHAD

CHAPTER 15

Das Mahavidya Yagna

Awake, arise!
Strive for the highest, and be in the light!
Sages say the path is narrow and difficult to tread,
Narrow as the edge of a razor."

— *Kathopanishad*

The invitation to Bharatpur was ostensibly to attend the *Das Mahavidya Yagna,* which was being held from 17th to 24th October, 2001. This coincided with the *Navratri* celebrations prior to *Durga Puja* or *Dussehra.* Early on 17th morning, I accompanied Pilot Baba to the temple where the *yagna* was being held. He personally checked the arrangements to ensure that all the preparations were satisfactorily completed.

Within the *shamiyana,* or temporary structure erected, the priests were busy preparing for the auspicious *yagna.* The antecedents of this *yagna* date a couple of millennia. Regarded as an extremely powerful *yagna,* it invokes ten forms of the Devi who are welcomed and appeased. Blessings are solicited and at the end of the period, the Devis are bade farewell with traditional respect for all rituals.

Yagnas are of different types, but only *satvik* or *vedic yagna,* which enjoys supremacy in the list of *yagnas,* should be performed. A *sadhak* of *satvik gunas* can always undo all *tantric kriyas* or activities. If he is a *yogi,* then the *tantrik* is more vulnerable to his powers. While Pilot Baba has spent time with Tibetan tantriks and is well versed in the nuances of the art, he is a *yogi*, who has remained steadfast on his path, and appeals to all t*antriks* to abstain from harmful practices, adding, "Every *tantrik* virtually stands on the verge of a painful death. Since he invokes Kali he can easily become her victim."

The *Das Mahavidya yagna* involves worship of ten aspects of Durga. She is worshipped first as Kali, the destroyer of the forces of evil, of enemies and of demons. She is invoked as Tara, the merciful and the goddess of plenty. As Tipusundari or Shodashi or Bala, she bestows wealth and beauty and holds the secrets of Sri Vidya. Bhuvaneshwari or Annapurana is the generous food bearing mother who rules agricultural produce and ensures rich harvests. In the form of Chinnamasta, she is the patron of children and of health. As Bhairavi she yields power to control fear and rules the nether regions. As the potent Dumavati she is the destroyer of enemies. Pitambara or Bagala wields power over the mind and provides the ability to discriminate. As Matangi, she brings godspeed to all actions. As Kamala, she brings wealth and controls financial destinies.

Every morning for three hours, with an elaborate performance of rituals, puja was offered. With a brief break for a *phalahari* meal, without cereals and lentils, the afternoon was devoted to ritualistic performances at a *havana*. In the evenings there were *satsanghas*, which lasted some three hours at which *sadhus* and *sants* shared their insights of the Way.

At that time, I had very little exposure to rituals and traditional worship. I enjoyed the Sanskrit recitations of *shlokas*, witnessed the power of meditation, sought to understand the significance of the rituals, watched the varied aspects of worship by the devout and participated in the oblations. I also used the time to practise being a witness and watched my unquestioning mind absorb the impressions created by ritualistic worship. The stillness of my mind allowed me to be aware of the energy generated by different vibrations.

On the first day of the *yagna*, Gorakh Baba sat beside Pilot Baba throughout the proceedings and participated in the oblations. I sat opposite them, beside the renunciate Kusum, at the large central *Havana kund*, from where I could easily witness and follow the rituals.

Vishvenrdra Singh, 16th Maharaja of Bharatpur and twice elected MP, and his wife, Divya Singh, also an erstwhile MP, participated in the opening *pujas*. Some 25-30 people sat around the *kund*. In the smaller surrounding *kunds*, there were 8-10 people each, mostly married couples, since all ritualistic worship is performed essentially for personal and social welfare and is part of a traditional social order.

Shastriji, who belongs to Kumaon, Uttarakhand, was the chief priest. He generally accompanies Pilot Baba to the various *yagnas* conducted by him. Other than a wealth of scriptural learning, Shastriji had many tales to tell. He recounted how he had once accompanied Gorakh Baba and Pilot Baba to the higher Himalayas, and claimed that by their meditation, they had caused the icy glacial waters to boil so they could cook a meal in it.

Shastriji led the recitations conducted by several pandits, including his only son, whom he lost in a road accident days after this *yagna*. The young man had exceptional knowledge of the Vedas, and I would often refer to him for explanations of the rituals. I enjoyed several meaningful conversations with him. Equally well-versed in computer sciences, he was a remarkable lad, whose absence I felt deeply at subsequent *yagnas*.

Chapter 16

Beyond Death

Lead me from the unreal to the Real,
From the dark delusion of ignorance
To the light of knowledge,
From death to immortality.

— *Brihadaranyaka Upanishad*

The Kathopanishad tells the tale of how Nachiketa attained immortality. A *Yagna* was performed by Nachiketa's father who was widely known for his knowledge, riches and generosity. He undertook a practice, which in its last phase, required that he give up everything including his entire wealth, possessions and even his ego. Nachiketa, a sincere young seeker, noticed that his father was not giving the best of his possessions away and mentioned it. Presuming that he would be given to an enlightened spiritual teacher, he asked his father to whom he would be given. His father grew agitated. When Nachiketa persisted with his question, his irritated father replied, "I give you to Death."

Nachiketa understood clearly that this did not imply suicide. He figured that he needed to understand the mystery of Death. Believed to be the first mortal, Yama is the ruler of Death. He presides over the ancestral regions and the interim regions before rebirth, including heaven and hell. It is Yama who greeted Nachiketa of the *Kathopanishad*, when he stood resolute at Death's door for 3 days and nights to ask the secrets of immortality. For having kept him waiting, Yama offered Nachiketa three boons.

For his first boon, Nachiketa asked that his father recognise him and welcome him when they should meet again. This refers to knowledge of earthly realms and essentially refers to the traditional belief that through dutiful behaviour, righteous worship and strong bonds we seek to remain connected from life to life to our ancestral lineage.

Nachiketa, who was a sincere seeker and who followed both the spirit and the letter of the scriptures was then granted his second boon, knowledge of the science of fire or *agni vidya*, that unveils the mystery of heaven and provides knowledge of the celestial realms.

The *Kathopanishad*, *Svetasvatara* and *Dhyanabindu Upanishads* provide insight to these. *Tantrik* scriptures of *Rudra Yamala* and *Svachchananda Tantra* provide studies of these techniques. Adepts of this science are rare and are found among the Nath tradition. They have mastered knowledge of the fire without and the fire within.

This knowledge however, does not provide enlightenment and a fully prepared student like Nachiketa would only be satisfied by the secrets of immortality that bring total freedom. The third boon sought by Nachiketa, was one that Yama was extremely reluctant to give. He promised all else including life in the celestial realms, but did not want to share that wisdom. Eventually he gave this knowledge to Nachiketa.

This knowledge is the Truth of the Upanishads. In the words of the Upanishads, it cannot be known through much learning, nor through the intellect and sacred teaching. It is reached by the chosen of Him, because they choose Him. To his chosen, His glory is revealed.

The light of the *Atman* is invisible, concealed in all beings. It is seen by the seers of the subtle, when their vision is keen and clear. The *Atman* is the flame that shines in a pure heart when it seeks *Brahman* or union with universal consciousness.

Brahman or the Spirit Supreme is not seen in the field of vision with mortal eyes. This Truth is known by the *Atman* when it reaches *Brahman*, the Spirit Supreme. *Brahman* or pure Spirit is the Immortal. Those who know Brahman know Immortality.

CHAPTRE 17

Flame becomes a Raging Fire

"Brahman is seen in a pure soul as in a mirror clear,
And also in the Creator's heaven as clear as light;
But in the land of shades as remembrances of dreams,
And in the world of spirits
As reflections in trembling waters."

— *Kathopanishad*

In the quiet afternoon, during a brief lull after lunch, I sat in the shady courtyard of the temple. Pilot Baba was not around. There were several *sadhus* sitting around, absorbed in their own contemplations. Gorakh Baba stood for a moment at the entrance, glancing around, before he set aside a chair and sat on it. Seeing him alone, I seized the opportunity to request permission to ask a few questions. He immediately acquiesced.

Without any preamble, I asked him, "Who are you?" He laughed immediately with the easy friendliness I remembered well.

"How can I tell you who I am?" he countered. "I cannot see my own face, as you cannot see yours. I can only see your face as you can see mine. We recognise ourselves when we see ourselves reflected as in a polished mirror. Judge a person by their words, their actions and their behaviour. We live in different realms at different times. Who we are is a factor of time. Sometimes, who we are shines forth like a flame that cannot be denied. The flame becomes a raging fire that none can stop. Only then are we recognised universally," he said.

The language of *yogis* breaks all barriers of conventional thinking and causes one to contemplate eternal truths.

Several *sadhus* started to gather around us as he spoke. He quickly walked out the door of the temple, but not without a quiet promise, "I will talk to you again."

I remembered that I had once read: "Sages of Baba Gorakh Nath's calibre are the word of God in flesh." Pilot Baba had confirmed to me that his *darshan* was blessing enough. I had sought his *darshan.* His presence was an affirmation of the infinite living I sought.

That evening, to signify the end of the day's ritualistic worship, I watched as Gorakh Baba took the conch shell in his hand. Raising his head to the endless skies, Gorakh Baba's call on the conch shell was the call of Shiva. Who was it a call to? Who heard that call? Who blew the conch shell? Is the knower and the known One?

The next morning, Pilot Baba said to me, "You can leave anytime you choose."

I confirmed to him, "I have spoken to Gorakh Baba."

BRIEF TIME MAGNIFIED

CHAPTER 18

Fellow Travellers

"There is a light that shines
Beyond all things on Earth, beyond us all,
Beyond the heaven, beyond the highest,
The very highest heavens.
This is the light that shines in our heart."

— *Chandogya Upanishad*

There were many people I met during my week's stay at Bharatpur. Hari Om, with whom I had been in touch on e-mail for several weeks, had dutifully kept me informed of Pilot Baba's programme. He is a serious, young software engineer, also responsible for Pilot Baba's website. We spent time discussing how Baba's message could be made accessible to a larger audience and how to meet the needs of Babaji's growing international discipleship that are keen to be in touch with his teachings and his programmes.

Eran, a Jewish-born disciple of Pilot Baba, at the time living in the U.S., had arrived with the express purpose of spending time with him during the *yagna.* On occasion, we would leave behind the dust and the growing crowds at the grounds and chat over a cup of tea at a nearby stall. Talking to Eran gave me an insight into the mindset of the international disciple. I learnt about Eran's life, his relationship with his *guru* and what it is like to be a foreigner in a distant land with alien customs that pull at your heartstrings. Being one of the few people there he could easily relate to, we forged a warm friendship based on our mutual appreciation for Pilot Baba's teachings and the growing heartfelt need to spread a message of peace and goodwill.

Sonal is a personable young woman who works for an NGO. I found the courage of her convictions and her strength of character, refreshing. Matter of fact and brutally honest with herself, she is a delight to interact with. Drawn early to a spiritual life, she had left home, braving opposition, to live in Baba's ashram near Nainital. Convinced that there was life outside the hermitage to which she had to return, she is now working on a water conservation project in Madhya Pradesh. In a gesture of affection and regard, she presented me with a book written by her mentor and guide at work.

Sunil also works on the same project as Sonal, and like her, is a disciple of Baba. I started talking to him in a car in which we were travelling a 10-minute distance. He had much to say and we talked right through the evening. He explained why he had left Mumbai to work in a village at considerably less salary. Pointing to his designer T-shirt, he said, "I don't need this in the village. There is nothing I can spend on there, so what I earn is more than what I need. It gives me great satisfaction to know that I am doing work that I enjoy which is useful for the rural people." He recited words he had once written that were outpourings of his soul. He explained, "The last time I met Babaji, there were tears in my eyes when I was leaving. How could I tell him that I wished more people could hear the wisdom of his words, that something were done to preserve what he says?"

There were many others I met there, like passengers on a brief journey, whose memories fade, but with whom I spent a moment of brief recognition and saw their souls reflected in their eyes.

CHAPTER 19

Consecrated Ground

"The Spirit in thee is like a river.
Its sacred bathing place is contemplation;
Its waters are truth; its banks are holiness;
Its waves are love.
Go to that river for purification:
Thy soul cannot be made pure by mere water."

— *Hitopadesha*

While the *yagna* was going on, simultaneously preparations were aground for the *samadhi sthal* beside it. A pit was dug. It was important that it were made to exact specifications. I noticed that Pilot Baba was very particular about the *samadhi sthal*, and treated it as consecrated ground. Which it was, as I realised in the time to follow.

I heard repeated requests to ensure that the pit and the awnings were properly designed. Baba himself was supervising it. In the evening *pravachan*, Ram Narayan Das, who had organised the *yagna*, announced that if anything were lacking in the arrangements, Babaji would cancel the *samadhi*. The next day, while sitting before the fire at the *yagna*, Pilot Baba sent for the *tamboowala*, who was responsible for the awnings. Despite repeated reminders, instructions were not being followed.

At another time, the man who became the sage Pilot Baba, would probably have been provoked to anger. However, Pilot Baba had long since gained total control of his temper. The fire beneath his words would have made anyone listen to him. "*Sadhu-santon ke baat nahin maante ho.*" (You do not heed the words of the sages).

Then came the blessing that the man sought, "*Bahut paise banaoge*" (You will make lots of money).

Babaji reminded him of an eternal truth. "*Par maroge.*" (But death is inevitable).

If the man had listened with his heart, he would have heard words of wisdom in what followed. If he listened from fear, he would have postponed knowledge of the Way. "*Aur veh paisa leke kahan jaoge*? " (Where will you go with that money?)

Any human being who heard his words should have been compelled to stop in his tracks and ask the question, "Why am I here?" Or perhaps, "Where will I go after this?" Pilot Baba stops people wherever they are and reminds them, in different ways, "What are you looking for? Seek that wisdom which alone brings everlasting joy."

He belongs to a lineage which can embrace death in life and return as an act of conscious will—the act of creating yourself anew, burning the accumulated *samskaras* of the past. That is the saffron that he wears—the true saffron of a *mahayogi*.

I had gone to him and to Gorakh Baba to say, "Tell me the secrets of eternity that you know. Share those secrets with me." They had both answered, "Go to Death's door and ask for those secrets. Only Death has the answer to them." Yet, they had also said, "You will be enlightened."

Those who continuously burn their *karma* in the fire of knowledge will be freed of their *karmic* attachments. They will receive God's Light at the time of leaving the body. It has been said, "For a sincere seeker, it is assured that Mahavtar Babaji or someone from that lineage will be there to usher them into the Infinite."

With that promise, it is only cowardice that prevents us from standing at Death's door with senses controlled, maintain one-pointed focus and ask the questions no one else can answer. Nachiketa represents one of those rare awakened seekers, who once having glimpsed the Truth, will pursue the understanding of it till he finds the answer. Any mortal, steadfast in his search, who meditates at death's door, will be granted a boon, as Nachiketa was. What boon do we want from Death? Have we asked ourselves what Knowledge we seek?

CHAPTER 20

Beyond the Veil

"When the soul is in silent quietness it arises
And leaves the body,
And reaching the Supreme Spirit finds there
Its body of light.
It is the land of infinite liberty where,
Beyond its mortal body, the Spirit of man is free."

— *Chandogya Upanishad*

Pilot Baba says, "If a man can control all functions of his body, he becomes immersed in *Brahma.* In *Samadhi,* a *yogi* separates the astral and causal bodies and wanders in the *Brahmanda.* When a *yogi* is in a state of *samadhi,* his body becomes lifeless and his thoughts assume a perfect balance. The various needs of practical life are suspended and he acquires a tremendous physical strength."

He explains, "The cognition of the astral world, releases him from desire to return to the material world. After close communion with the creator's wondrous waves, he loses interest in the physical world. He rises above the limitations of the physical world. The creative impulse in man gives birth to desires and its consequent motion. A *yogi*'s life is devoid of *karma* and duty."

Baba explains, "A *yogi* who is on the plane of cosmic consciousness can comprehend all the activities of the *Brahmanda,* which appear in the form of astral vibrations. By virtue of his astral knowledge, he detaches himself from revealed nature, goes deep within the Self and wanders in the folds of eternity. By renouncing the intellect, mind, ego,

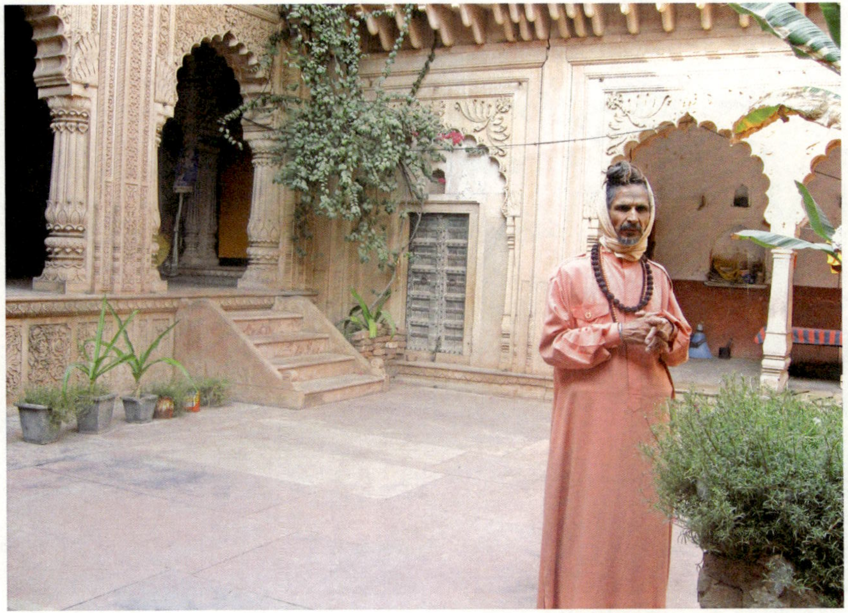

GORAKH BABAJI - AT MANDIR AT BHARATPUR

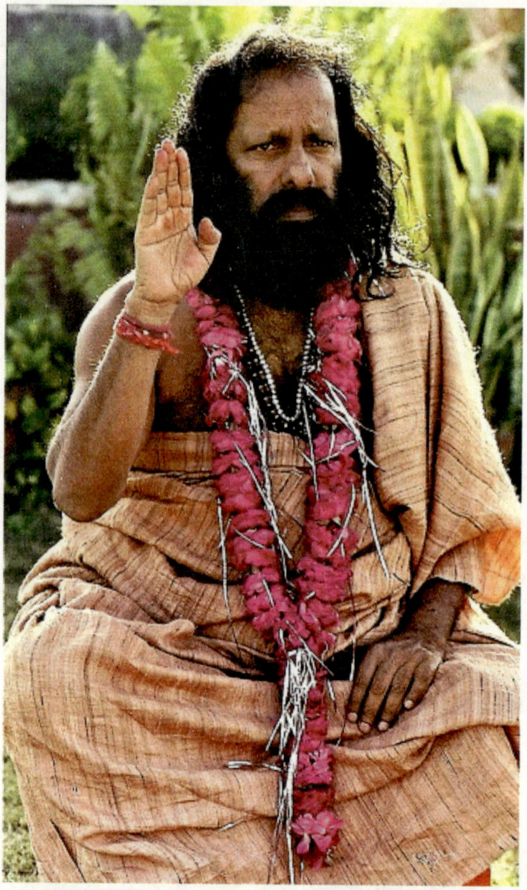

PILOT BABAJI - A QUIET MOMENT

chit, a *yogi* obtains the propensity to rise towards the *Tejas* or Supreme Intelligence. Saints and *mahatmas* who have freed themselves from the worldliness of life, can obtain this level of *samadhi.* A Self-illumined *yogi* is free from birth and death."

Referring to the *samadhi* taken by sages, he says, "Generally, a *mahapurush* takes *samadhi* in the security of caves and secluded places. He then enjoys the astral world for long periods."

He asserts, "A *samadhi* is not a trivial issue and should not be undertaken for the sake of trial or exhibition." It becomes imperative that the sanctity of a *samadhi* is maintained. When Pilot Baba, or one of his disciples, takes *samadhi* in public view, it is taken with the express *sankalpa* of fostering peace, love and harmony.

Pilot Baba has been responsible for several of his disciples taking *sthal samadhi* in public view. They are all clearly aware that they take *samadhi* with the *guru's shakti.* The state of *samadhi* is an inert state of the body and the mind. There are several levels of *samadhi.* Sages immemorial, have immersed themselves in deep meditation that leads to *samadhi. Samadhi* is not the same as enlightenment and Baba repeats again and again, "No one else can give you enlightenment. Recognise yourself and you will be enlightened."

CHAPTER 21

Astral Journeys

" Meditation is in truth higher than thought.
The earth seems to rest in silent meditation;
And the waters and the sky and the heavens
Seem all to be in meditation."

— *Chandogya Upanishad*

Chandra had been preparing for her *samadhi* for a long time. When I was first introduced to her, she was already immersed in her preparation for it. Chetna was her constant companion. Chetna and Chandra are sisters in all but birth. They have a perfect rapport of love, sharing and trust that can sometimes be seen among siblings. Chetna had already taken *samadhi* three times.

Chandra was on a reduced diet of milk and soup. The last couple of days were spent in isolation, and her nutrition intake was totally withdrawn on the last day. The evening before her *samadhi*, Baba blessed her, after which no one was supposed to disturb her meditative state. Even the slightest touch could awaken her unpleasantly.

The crowds had gathered from early morning. The *samadhi sthal* was barricaded off to keep the crowds at a reasonable distance. Repeated announcements on the mike said that no one should attempt to touch her when she came to the *sthal* as it could result in bodily harm to the person touching her. Chants of *'Om Namoh Shivay'* now rent the air in a wave of devotion that enveloped the space.

Just after noon, Yogmata Shraddha, as Chandra now was, came in Baba's jeep. In his official capacity as

Mahamandaleshwar or a leader of the Juna Akhara, the largest sect of Indian *sadhus,* Baba's vehicle has a distinctive emblem. The vehicle drove up to the cordoned off area and she emerged and stood on a platform before the thousands of waiting devotees, believers and spectators, before sitting in the public gaze and waiting for the scheduled time of 1 p.m., when she would go into *samadhi.*

The pit was now covered with tin sheeting, tarpaulin and earth, except for an opening through which she would descend by a ladder, sit on a wooden bench and meditate for about a minute before going into *samadhi* at 1 sharp. Once inside, the opening would be sealed off with tin, tarpaulin and mounds of earth.

Today the empty pit had a *trishul,* the colour of gold. Mahayogi Kapil Advait, fondly nicknamed Pilot Baba, descended into the pit. Yogmata Shraddha was ready to go into the bowels of the earth. Completely calm and serene, there was not a flicker of any kind of thought reflected on her face. As she was getting ready to descend, an enthusiastic onlooker threw a garland that fell across her neck. Yogmata Shraddha's face became suffused with colour. The Mahayogi's reaction was instantaneous. He threw the garland off and absorbed the effects of this disturbance onto himself. Turning to Yogmata Shraddha, he blessed her by placing his hand above her shoulder. Her face relaxed immediately and the calm returned.

The Mahayogi stood watching, as she stepped down the ladder, stepped onto the wooden plank and touched the hundreds of *rudraksha malas* placed by devotees for blessing. She quickly settled into her *asana.* Keeping a strict eye on his watch, Pilot Babaji raised his hand in blessing and the pit was sealed off. Before the last mounds of earth were thrown in, he peeped in once, before giving the signal to seal off the pit. Later, Chetna and Kusum made a simple decoration of rice and flowers to mark the space.

Three days and nights, Yogmata Shraddha remained in *samadhi.* Devotees and disciples came in thousands to pay their homage outside the barricades of the site. Within it, at all times, there were one, two or more of Baba's close associates who kept vigil. Throughout the day, several people sat just outside, keeping a watch. During the nights, several *sadhus* kept protective vigil at the *samadhi sthal.*

The first evening, we spent a wonderful time bonding, while chatting with Chetna about her *samadhi* experiences at different times and places. Kusum, Chetna, Hari Om, Eran and I sat talking while people continued with their *parikrama* around the *sthal* and crowds listened to the speeches made by various *sadhus* in the *pandal* earmarked for the *pravachan.*

Chetna explained that every time she had taken *samadhi,* it had always been undertaken with a particular *sankalpa.* The *samadhi* undertaken by Yogmata Shraddha was for world peace. Chetna said that she went into *samadhi* by an act of will, mastered through the practice of particular *kriyas.* She explained that during the *samadhi,* one literally leaves one's body and moves in one's astral form. Returning to the body involves allowing your soul consciousness to enter the physical body — a practice she undertakes with the *guru's shakti,* purely at his instance.

Eran asked, "What does Pilot Baba himself do when he has to return from his own *samadhi?*"

Chetna replied, "He is already well-versed in the practice. His *guru* must have given him the required instruction."

Someone wanted to know what happens if your *samadhi* breaks before the time allotted. Chetna replied with total faith and surrender, "The disciple remains connected to the *guru,* who protects you, throughout the *samadhi.*"

Referring to a particular instance during one of her *samadhis,* she recalled suddenly thinking, "My body has started breathing." She became instantly afraid, adding that there are disembodied spirits with evil intentions who seek to embody themselves. As soon as she grew aware of her own mind and body and began to respond to her thoughts she felt the protective influence of her *gurudev,* Pilot Babaji. She knew that no harm could befall her. Instantly, her fear subsided and she could again witness her lifeless body at rest while she remained in *samadhi,* till the appointed time.

Chapter 22

Face of Suffering

"When selfishness and violence and pride are gone;
When lust and anger and greed are no more;
Free from the thought 'this is mine'
A man rises to the mountain of the highest,
Worthy to be one with Brahman, with God"

—*Bhagavad Gita*

While Yogmata Shraddha remained in *samadhi*, there were continuous crowds who thronged the barricades that shielded the *samadhi sthal*. They did *parikrama*, 3 times, 21 times, 108 times, each according to his faith and his worship. They came in curiosity, they arrived for *darshan* of the *samadhi sthal*, they offered worship, they sought peace, they came to pray for solutions to their problems, they asked the gods to fulfil their desires. Some came in silence, others chanted, '*Om Namoh Shivay*', several of them prostrated themselves, while many came with folded hands. A few stood still and watched.

Sitting at the *samadhi sthal* for a large part of the three days, I sought to be a witness to it all. One day, it seemed to me that the extent of human suffering was seemingly more than I wanted to cope with. I watched people come to Baba for his blessings. Each came with a problem. He remained completely detached, even when he offered solace.

When he was not there, they continued to arrive seeking absolution. Distress writ large on her face, a woman came with a disturbed young son who was constantly violent and abusive. A young girl came whose sister had committed suicide and her brother had died soon after. A child of eight said she was very unhappy because her father beat her mother and her every day. A woman came saying her husband is unfaithful and she cannot cope with her own jealousies. An obviously psychotic woman wept copious tears. A woman who could neither hear nor speak gesticulated her agony. They came in droves and poured out their suffering.

The dust raised from the hundreds of feet that were circumambulating the *samadhi sthal* was almost unbearable. I sat there listening to a renunciate asking, "What am I doing here? I had not come for this. When I return home, I no longer belong there either." I decided I needed to take a walk.

As I stepped out on to the road and started walking, I felt alone with myself, after several days. I walked that road as though it was the road of my life, and in the short distance I tread the path of an unknown town, alone with myself, I saw my entire life slipping behind me and I walked as though completely lost. I walked as in the last moments of life, when you review your life as in a reel of film, and you have no option then of shutting it off, rewinding or fast forwarding. The film is canned and you can only observe it. I was aware of the words, "Nothing belongs to you."

I had not noticed the old sage in white, staff in hand, who approached me from the other side. I stood before him and gazed deep into his eyes, as only the truly fearless or the truly lost, can do. And my eyes filled with tears. As they almost had, when I met Gorakh Baba recently. My voice had broken when I spoke to him about twelve years of living with a single sentence.

When I spoke to Pilot Baba on the phone after long years he had said, "You have not heard my voice in a long time. How are you?" I had answered "Very well," but my voice betrayed emotion.

But now, caught unaware by an old unknown *sadhu*, my tears flowed. He said, "*Yeh kasht kyon*?" (Why this suffering?) The silent tears flowed down my cheeks. "*Himmat nahin harna,* "(You must not lose courage), he said, and shaking his head admonished me firmly, "*Aaj ke baad kabhi nahin ro'oge.*" (You will never cry again). But I was quite inconsolable, though I was bereft of speech.

Suddenly, he became nurturing, "*Kasht karna hamara kaam hota hai.*" (Suffering is our work) And then, with the power of sages to grant a boon, he said, "*Apna kasht hame de do.*" (Give me your suffering). With that, he placed his hand on my head in benediction, to take on himself my suffering, born surely of my own *karmas.*

As he removed his hand, he said, "*Hamare liye kasht kar rahe ho*?" (You are suffering for us?) And with great sadness, he shook his head, saying, "*Nahin*" (no). And before I knew it, he had bent to touch my feet, saying, "*Yeh bhav ko pranam kar raha hoon.*" (I acknowledge your feeling).

We both walked on in opposite directions. I knew my courage had been restored. I had learnt the lesson Pilot Baba had tried to explain to me about the nature of suffering and how to detach oneself from it. Later, every time I saw suffering, whether my own or that of someone else, I tried to remind myself, "It is their own *karma.*"

I had realised that my own suffering was of my own creation. That I have known much joy is also my *karma.* I decided to view life, as I always had, as a master who bestows knowledge, as both Gorakh Baba and Pilot Baba had advised. Pilot Baba had said, "You will not have a *guru.* Let life be your teacher. Learn from everyone you meet."

I felt certain I would find the answers to all the questions I have sought.

Chapter 23

Return to the World

"He who knows both the transcendent and the immanent,
With the immanent overcomes death,
And with the transcendent reaches immortality."

— *Chandogya Upanishad*

Exactly seventy-two hours from the time that Yogmata Shraddha went into *samadhi,* she was due to return to the world. The crowds were almost frenzied in their attempt to reach the *samadhi sthal.* The barricades erected now kept them further at bay. The police, batons on display, controlled the crowds.

The crowds within the barricade of the *samadhi sthal* were growing continuously, because several of Ram Narayan Das's disciples had been permitted in. The press had been given entry and press photographers and cameramen were jostling to get the best view. There were various other people who had also entered the area.

Outside the crowds were getting noisier in their eagerness for *darshan.* In preparation for her emergence to the world of lights, noise and people, the earth was being removed by hand by some of Baba's disciples, without stepping on the immediate pit. Suddenly an elderly man ran on top of the pit and started removing the earth. Baba bent down to pick a handful of earth and threw it at the man to make him beat a hasty retreat. It was another instance I saw of Baba's adherence to sanctity of this consecrated ground. When he noticed that some people were wearing their slippers, he turned them out instantly. However, he did not object when they returned without their footwear.

Baba stood guarding the pit, looking at his watch at intervals. At the appropriate time, he bent, removed the tarpaulin and lifted a tin sheet slightly, to peep in. He raised a thumbs-up sign, completely uncharacteristic of his usual gestures. I smiled at this glimpse of his personality.

The tarpaulin and tin sheets were removed from overhead so Baba could descend into the pit. A ladder was placed. He descended and stood beside Yogmata Shraddha, who sat in *samadhi.* He placed his hand over her head. Instantly, she rubbed her eyes exactly as Baba instructs at the end of a meditation. Her hands automatically went to Baba's feet as she bowed before him. She stood up and climbed the ladder out of the pit. Another ladder raised her onto the platform where people were queuing to receive her *darshan.*

The crowds were almost uncontrollable. I desperately sought an exit. I sat awhile in the tent where Baba's *trishul* was placed. I walked out and returned to where I was staying. A few hours later, I sat with Chetna, Kusum, Sonal and Shraddha as they enjoyed their meal. The late afternoon was spent reclining awhile immersed in conversations. In the evening, Sunil and a couple of others joined in. It was one of those rare occasions when we all sat with Baba in his room, relaxing, chatting, laughing.

The next morning, on sudden impulse, I decided to go to Vrindavan for a day, on my way to Delhi and Kolkata, before returning to Mumbai. Baba placed his hand on my head in blessing and gave me *prasad.* His customary words of parting to me are exactly what I have always told my son in parting. They convey an abiding affection, concern and protection, "Take care of yourself."

At Kolkata, I had a relaxed and immensely enjoyable holiday with my family. Rajiv joined us there. My brother, Rahul and I had always been very close. My parents were thrilled to have both their children and their son-in-law and daughter-in-law with them, at the same time. It was the last time. Barely a couple of months after Rahul returned to the US, he lost his life in a car accident.

The last e-mail from him was accessed by me after I had learnt that he had already gone, and in it, he had written, in the context of the death of a friend of his, "Life continues as usual." Yes, indeed, I do believe that life continues, in many different realms and spaces, where we can always easily connect, in silence and through our feelings.

My brother's joy at my pleasures was unbound, his pride at my smallest achievement was touching, he always reached out to offer comfort and support when he thought I was in any way upset. Equally, there was no aspect of his life that I was not aware of or that he did not readily share. And yet, we were not embroiled in each other's lives. I would like to believe that we loved each other very completely and without attachment.

One of the last mails I had exchanged with him was about an esoteric treatise, conducted in the form of questions from Gorakh Nath to Matsyendra Nath, that we had both been moved by. There were many questions and to each there was an answer.

"Had there been no body, where would the spirit have been?"

"Without the body, the spirit would have been in the Supreme Void."

"Which is the door of the Void?"

"Realisation is the door of the Void."

SHIVA

CHAPTER 24

Legends of Shiva

"Give thy mind to me, and give me thy heart,
And thy sacrifice, and thy adoration.
This is my word of promise:
Thou shalt in truth come to me, for thou art dear to me."

— *Bhagavad Gita*

Every Indian has already formed an idea of Shiva, mainly from images and symbols of him and from anecdotes we may have heard. Shiva is liberally depicted in the art forms of poetry and dance. He is the creator of dance through his *Rudra Tandava* in anger and *Ananda Tandava* in joy. From his *damaru* comes the *Akṣarasamāmnāya*, or 14 rhythmic syllables from which Panini compiled and codified the rules of Sanskrit Grammer. His temples are everywhere. His association through his symbols are also well represented. The undeniable presence of the *yogis* of India is a reminder of those who aspire to know and understand what Shiva represents.

One of the three aspects of the Hindu Trinity of Brahma the Creator, Vishnu the Preserver and Mahesh the Destroyer, Shiva is the most commonly used of 1008 names to denote him. Other names include Mahadeva, the great God; Rudra, the early Vedic god; Neelkanth, the blue-throated One; and Ishwara, the Supreme. As the destroyer of all evil, he is believed to take the world through its cycle of cosmic dissolution into the next phase of creation.

As the legends of the Ramayana and the Mahabharata have been brought to us by the sages, Valmiki and Vyas, the legends of Shiva have been handed down by the sages to express an awareness of the realms where Shiva resides. His abode is Mount Kailash in the Himalayas. He is the perfect family man. His eternal consort is depicted as manifesting and returning to him in different lifetimes in different forms. This aspect of his life as a bridegroom is envisioned by poets, writers, painters and in dance form.

Lord Shiva is depicted as a dark-skinned blue-throated ascetic with matted hair, covered with the ashes of cremation grounds, seated in meditation on a tiger skin. He wears a garland of *rudraksha* beads, when he is envisioned as the meditating ascetic. A garland of flowers depicts his benevolent playful aspect. The garland of skulls shows his *tapasya* form, a reminder of Devi's manifestation from life to life. Vasuki, the Naga king, signifies protection. The *damaru* represents primordial sound from which time and space are created. His *trishul* signifies the ultimate weapon of protection of the forces of good; and of destruction of the forces of evil. The *kamadhenu*, or ascetic's bowl, symbolises austerity. The clarion call on the conch shell is the call of Lord Shiva. The raised hand is the blessing and protection that he gives.

Lord Shiva is not a worldly god, munificent in his distribution of largesse. Worship of Lord Shiva is not bound to the many legends, rituals and festivals that are usually associated with worship of Lord Vishnu in his main *avatars* of Rama and Krishna, who have their obvious appeal as readily approachable gods with a human face. Brahma worship is relatively rare. Envisioned as a mother, the Devis are commonly worshipped, easier to appease and readily grant worldly desires.

Shiva is envisioned as the boatman in Benaras, where he crosses devotees across the sea of *samsara* by reciting the *Taraka mantra*. He is depicted as a wanderer of cremation grounds among funeral pyres. He is worshipped alike by those who worship the forces of light and those who worship the forces of darkness. There are many esoteric cults and unconventional methods of offering worship to Lord Shiva. There are several forms of *Tantrik* worship that are also dedicated to him.

Sati's choice of bridegroom at a *swayamvara* when she garlands Shiva, the wandering ascetic, who walks in, is an oft-told tale. Her sacrificial death when her husband is still treated as an outcaste by her father, Daksha when she visits her parental home, and the ensuing mad grief of Shiva at losing her, is legendary. All the gods, including Vishnu, desperately appease him to calm him down. Lord Shiva goes into deep meditation and is not even aware when she returns as Parvati, daughter of the Himalayas, who meditates and undertakes great penances before he acknowledges her.

It is said that his third eye opened when Parvati playfully covered his eyes with her hands while he was in meditation. Immediately, the universe was plunged into darkness and there was chaos. To reinstate order, a fire emitted from his forehead and restored light to the world. This is Lord Shiva's third eye, which oversees the world at all times and also has the power to destroy.

Once both the gods and demons decided to churn the oceans to extract the ambrosia of life. While the gods chanted *mantras* and performed ritual oblations for the sacred venture, the demons arrived intent on drinking the very nectar of life.

In the ensuing battle for supremacy between the gods and the demons, the oceans started spilling out a lethal poison that threatened to overcome the world. To save the world, Shiva consumed the poison, containing it in his throat. The poison turned Lord Shiva's throat blue and accounts for his name, Neelkantha.

There is a legend about sage Narada, disciple of Narayana who visited Shiva's ashram at Mount Kailash. Finding Shiva away at Badrinath, Narada who was intent on benefiting mankind by revealing the well-concealed secrets of eternity, presented a morose and abject face to Parvati. On her insistence to know the cause of his sadness, Narada told her he was grieved by the extent of deception in the world, and inconsolable at seeing the same betrayal by Shiva himself. Parvati would not believe it, but Narada cleverly pointed out to her, "Shiva does not love you as much as he claims he does. What he values most he has not shared with you."

At Parvati's insistence that Narada explain himself, he asked quietly, "Mother, whose skulls does Shiva wear as a garland around his neck?"

Parvati exclaimed, "He loves me so much that in my remembrance he preserves my skull every time I leave my body."

Narada replied, "So he has not shared with you the secrets of Immortality that he himself knows?"

When Shiva returned home, a visibly distressed Parvati had to be cajoled into explaining her hurt. "Why have you not told me the secrets of immortality?" she asked eventually.

Shiva laughed, "Because you had not asked for it. I will tell you now. The only condition is that no one else should hear it."

As Shiva sat to unfold the mysteries to Parvati, Narada devised a complicated and convoluted plan to overhear the secrets through the sage Sukh Deva, who was in hiding. Shiva discovering Sukh Deva, raised his *trishul* to kill him, but Brahma Rishi Vyasa, already immortal by Shiva's decree, stood in protection of his son, Sukh Deva, while Narada and Narayana arrived to remind Shiva of his protection of Vyasa. A laughing Shiva withdrew his trident.

CHPATER 25

Master of Ascetics

"I am the Way,
And the Master who watches in silence;
Thy friend and thy shelter and thy abode of peace.
I am the beginning
And the middle and the end of all things:
Their seed of eternity,
Their treasure Supreme."

— *Bhagavad Gita*

Shiva is the lord and master worshipped by ascetics. He is the *guru* of the immortal sages. They have sought to understand the secrets of the Universe from Shiva who stands beyond the doors of birth and death. Matsyendra Nath received the secret teachings of immortality from him. His eternal disciple, Guru Gorakh Nath has, for centuries untold, guided disciples towards the eternal truths that bring enlightenment. Pilot Baba was spiritually awakened by Hari Baba.

Shiva can only be known through intense meditation. Himself immersed in meditation, Shiva is neither involved in, nor does he interfere with the usual course of events. He remains indifferent and detached from worldly affairs. Even though he is known as the destroyer, Shiva is not concerned with mortal death.

In the world of man he walks past unnoticed. Addressed as *Mahayogi*, or the great ascetic, he symbolises the highest form of austere penance and abstract meditation, the ultimate goal of which is union with cosmic consciousness.

Sometimes he stands before us in his ascetic form to remind us of the Infinite path we walk unconsciously.

The living who seek death in order to understand and go beyond death to an eternal life, meet Shiva in the spaces where he walks. He sees the depth of human misery and remains completely detached because he knows he has the power to re-create the world at Will. When good and evil cannot be judged by common man, Shiva comes then to destroy evil. When the weapons of destruction that have been amassed are enough to annihilate the world, Shiva stands in protection of a sacred space.

CHAPTER 26

Call of Shiva

**"Go to him for thy salvation with all thy soul.
By his grace thou shalt obtain the peace supreme,
Thy home of Eternity."**

— *Bhagavad Gita*

I had been clearly told by Pilot Baba not to look for gods. "They do not exist", were Baba's words to me. I replied that I had never believed in them, not realising that I had chanted, '*Aum Namoh Shivay*'. The first time I had done so was at Patal Bhuvaneshwar in the Kumaon Himalayas, where we had gone 12 years earlier on Baba's recommendation.

It was dark and we were entering the bowels of the earth in a cave where sages, it is believed, had meditated through the centuries. The priest, who was entering at the time, advised the chant of '*Aum Namoh Shivay.*' When I repeated the words for the first time in my life, I knew it was one of many *mantras* I knew unconsciously. At the time, my fear had disappeared. Since then, sometimes in the conquest of fear, I have chanted the *mantra.* I have generally meditated with '*Aum*'. More often than not, I have meditated without any *mantra.*

Baba had now said, "The gods do not exist". Having forgotten that I had invoked Shiva, I readily denied the gods. He said to me, "Even God does not exist. Go beyond That."

I had always believed that God exists. I created a formless image of God in my mind as a child. I related to a personal God with whom I could always commune without any barriers. God was totally protective. My faith and trust were unshakeable.

As I grew older, the Upanishads gave me an intellectual awareness of non-duality, which appealed to my rational mind. God spoke to me of Eternal Truths in an Eternity of Time. I acknowledged anyone through whom these words of wisdom manifested, as a messenger of Truth.

One day, sitting in meditation, I was completely unaware that I had gone into a state of deep meditation. I had forgotten to take the *sankalpa* Baba had advised me to take—that of time. I had been instructed to set myself a time before I went into deep meditation. "Just before you go into that darkness," Baba had reminded me. I should have realised the impossibility of that statement. I went through the door into darkness without fear, intent as I was on my search.

I had already been given the blessings of Pilot Baba and Gorakh Baba. I had their protection, though I was not conscious of it. I went into the darkness without awareness of myself. Through that darkness, I grew aware of the presence of Shiva. I was almost annoyed at being disturbed. I did not want any miracles or appearances. Enough sages were now guiding me towards the understanding I sought. I could recognise them clearly.

When Shiva came, I had no difficulty recognising him though he came in thought waves, not in form. Shiva stood before me and reminded me that I had called. I replied, "Then it was so long ago, I don't remember."

He asked me what boon I wanted from him. Anyone whose call Shiva answers is granted a boon. Attracting Shiva's attention is to wake him from his deep *samadhi* and endure his wrath to seek eternal truths. I said, "What boon should I ask of you, who has come in your eternal form to one who is limited by a mortal form?"

I told him that I had sought knowledge and wisdom. I had sought Eternal Truths. When I recognised the sages through the Truths they spoke, I had acknowledged them. I had asked for Truth. They had sent me to Shiva. Or Shiva had come to me of his own volition. I reminded him that he had not shared with me the Eternal Truths I had sought.

In silence, he turned to leave. I knew he would answer me eventually. I asked for his *trishul* for protection as he left.

I knew the power of Shiva's *trishul.* I had seen Baba's *trishul* placed in protection during the period of *samadhi.* I first saw it in the empty pit, and knew it was the ultimate weapon of protection. I had touched the *trishul* while placing it away, after the *samadhi.* I knew I had to ask Shiva for his weapon of defence, because then I would be protected.

Later still, completely focused and alert with senses, mind, body and consciousness in a state of awareness, I performed a symbolic offering of my life. My meditation was a vocal prayer that I had spontaneously learned while meditating.

I invoked Shiva, saying, "Come, stand beside me as I sit in meditation. Let the power of your *trishul* be my protection".

I was determined that no matter who came and stood in front of me, I would not recognise them until I had recognised myself.

And then I prayed, "Into the river of time, I offer my union with this life. Shiva is my witness."

"Into the winds I scatter the beauty, joys, love and perfection of this life as I have known it."

"Into the fire, I offer my *samskaras,* so that nothing remains of me."

"May the forces of good triumph over the forces of evil."

"May the seed of *sankalpa* which created this play of consciousness be dissolved, so the pure light of consciousness shines forth."

It was a symbolic offering. I offered myself. For the Eternal Truths I had sought.

I knew the world of living well. I could leave it behind without looking at it.

I had to pass through the celestial realms without stopping. I had sought the protection of Shiva's *trishul*—Shiva, the ascetic mendicant. For this foray into the Infinite, He was bound to protect me, even against himself. I met no one at all.

When I emerged on the other side, I knew I had crossed the fires. I was aware that henceforth I could call on the elements for their protection. I had prayed to them daily for their cooperation—to the earth, the fires, the winds, the waters and all of nature.

I knew that I was not the body and I was not the mind. I was the Self Beyond.

I stood at other doors. I passed through the world of spirits, and did not look left or right. There were many there. I remained detached. I walked on aware of the illusory nature of the realm.

And then I came to those worlds I have inhabited and saw the people whom I knew, living different lives. They could not see me. When I called out, they could not hear. I travelled in astral form and saw different realms coexist. Not entirely without pain. I knew that pain had made me forget past existences. I was no longer willing to forget, if it meant that I would also forget the Wisdom that came with the living.

I returned to my body and to this life without noticing the transition. I had not noticed a transition when leaving either. I had walked into an eternity I was already familiar with. I had sought that eternity.

I was aware that I had returned my body to the elements in more lives than one. I have lived in other realms of existence. If I stayed focused, constantly alert, awakened and aware, I would be able to leave my body in consciousness.

I returned in search of a purpose higher than myself. The only purpose I have sought in my life. Those Eternal Truths that cause one to return in silence. And then try to express them so they can be shared.

Epilogue

"Glory be to that God who is in the fire,
Who is in the waters,
Who is in plants and trees,
Who is in all things in this vast creation.
Unto that spirit be glory and glory."

— *Svetasvatara Upanishad*

Guru Gorakh Nath said, "Shame on the aspirant who claims to be sincere but dies without accomplishing the purpose of life. And shame on the teacher who claims to be a *sadguru* if his disciple dies before reaching the goal." An enlightened master may have many followers and devotees but he rarely accepts a disciple. Once he has accepted a disciple he is committed to guide him all the way to enlightenment, through lifetimes of living, if need be. It becomes his commitment to hasten the process of enlightenment.

I have sought the guidance of the masters whom I have met and recognised. Although I am not an initiated disciple of anyone, I am well aware that both Gorakh Baba and Pilot Baba have given me their ultimate blessings and total protection, which a *guru* usually only bestows on his chosen disciples. Pilot Baba assured me, "You will be enlightened." Gorakh Baba reaffirmed, "You will find all the answers." In all humility, I acknowledge their blessings and protection.

When I went for the *yagna* at Bharatpur, after the *ahuti*, Pilot Baba placed a *tika* on my forehead. This has customarily to be accepted with *guru dakshina*. Observing everyone else, I offered money, but he shook his head.

At a *yagna* at Pipariya, watching everyone else, I was unsure of what to do. I reached into the pocket of my jeans and Pilot Baba clearly said, "not necessary". The next day, as he got up to lead the ritual bath of the invoked Devi and of Ganesh, he told me in passing, to keep sitting. I sat and watched worshippers feverishly bathe and clothe the goddess in symbolic appeasement. I found myself saddened as I silently addressed the goddess, "They will invoke you, but they will not respect you". Almost immediately, Pilot Baba's voice admonished the crowds of worshippers, "Worship the one you invoke. Whatever you do, must be done with respect."

After the final symbolic offering into the fires of the *Havana kund*, along with everyone else, I went to Pilot Baba for the *trilok tika* he was bestowing. I accepted it with bowed head and folded hands. The day I was leaving Pipariya, I went to receive the *trilok tika.* I closed my eyes and lowered my head in acknowledgement. I felt the blessing of the *trishul* when Pilot Baba touched three fingers to my forehead, forcibly raising my head, and silently saying that the way ahead was not of humility alone, but that I would have to exercise the strength, courage, determination and discrimination to use the powers that I could invoke. It was a reminder that Shiva protects me.

I must remain aware that I now move through the world, without saffron robes, protected by the fires. I pray continuously that the fires, the earth, the air, the waters and all of nature cooperate with me.

I tread the spaces of the immortal masters with their blessings. In ascetic wandering I have traversed through the Himalayas alone, meditating in the footsteps of the *rishis* of old: Vashishtha, Vyas, Bhrigu. I have met sages untold. I have followed the Panch Kedar trail where the Pandavas performed austerities seeking Shiva's *darshan* to free themselves from the killings of the Mahabharata to attain immortal light.

I have sought Shiva's protection so that I may learn to meditate as long as it takes to be heard by him. May my vision be purified so that I can be a seer of the subtle and stand in the immortal spaces where Shiva lives and ask him yet again for the secrets of immortality that he has long denied me.

"*Aum*
This eternal word is all:
What was, what is and what shall be,
And what beyond is in eternity.
All is *Aum*."

— *Mandukya Upanishad*

Glossary

Advaita : non-dualism.

Ahuti : offering, oblation. Any solemn rite accompanied with oblation.

Ananda : bliss, the unadulterated joy of pure being.

Asanas : postures that strengthen the body and sharpen the mind; practised for the purpose of achieving one-pointedness.

Ashram : hermitage. A secluded abode for study and spiritual practice.

Atman : the true or higher self as distinct from the ego- conscious self. The permanent essence and individualised super-consciousness. The non- individualised supreme consciousness is Paramatma.

Aum : primal sound or vibration from which the universe emanates. The sacred sound and symbol which represents Brahman.

Aum Namoh Narayana : Aum, thy name is Narayana, a mantra saluting Vishnu.

Aum Namoh Shivaya : Aum thy name is Shiva, a mantra saluting Shiva as the higher self.

Avatar : incarnation of the divine in human form.

Baba : an affectionate term meaning "father", used for a guru or a holy man. Many venerated saints are referred to as Baba or Babaji. The Ji is a suffix denoting respect.

Benaras : ancient city now known as Varanasi.

Bhagwati : one of the names of the Universal Mother.

Brahman : absolute or Ultimate Reality. The One Absolute Being from whom everything emanates.

Brahmanda : universe, cosmos.

Buddhi : root—*budh*, to know. Knowledge and the faculty of discernment.

Chandra : moon.

Chetna : literally, awareness.

Chit : pure undifferentiated consciousness.

Dalmoth : snacks.

Damaru : small drum varying in length from 6 to 12 inches. Associated with Lord Shiva who plays this instrument when he dances the tandava nritya. The drum is shaped like an hour-glass with two skin heads laced to the body by a thread.

Darshan : literally, to see; direct experience. To have darshan of a guru refers to the insight gained from a manifestation of divinity.

Dhuni : a sacred smouldering fire, tended by ascetics.

Diksha : spiritual initiation.

Gorakh : literally meaning a person who has mastered his senses (indriyas) and has complete control over the five vikritis (negative qualities) in human nature, namely kaam (sexual impulses), krodh (anger), lobh (greed), moh (attachment) and madh (ego).

Gufa : cave.

Gunas : the three aspects or qualities of the manifest Godhead and of Prakriti. Sattva being the force of truth, harmony, purity. Rajas is the tendency towards power, desire and energy. Tamas, the inclination towards inertia and stagnation. When the Gunas were in disequilibria, the godhead manifested the known universe.

Guru : literally that which dispels darkness. Spiritual teacher. Often this relationship is cemented when a guru initiates a disciple into meditation. The sadguru or satguru (enlightened master) commits to guide his disciple all the way to enlightenment, through lifetimes of living if need be.

Guru Dakshina : ritualistic offering given by a disciple to his Guru/teacher.

Guru Purnima : day reserved for homage to the Guru. A festival, related to the element of Spirit. Occurs in late July or early August.

Havan Kunda : sacrificial pit.

Jal Samadhi : see Samadhi.

Jiva/Jeeva : individualised soul.

Karma : root–*kri*, to act, do or make. A completed action. Actions, though com-plete, exist in subtle form in the un-conscious mind and theresult of the karma will manifest sooner or later.

		The law of Karma, or causality, states that samskaras(subtle impressions) dictate our actions. Action in turn creates fresh samskaras, thus leaving us trapped inthe vicious circle of causality with no free will. Karmas can be beneficial or negative and are categorised as:
Sanchita	:	stored or dormant.
Prarabdha	:	active.
Kriyamana	:	potential.
		Only by breaking the cycle of Karma can we master our own destiny.
Karmic	:	Pertaining to Karma.
Kathopanishad or Katha-Upanishad	:	a part of the Yajur Veda. Depicting an interaction between the ideal student and the ultimate teacher, it narrates how a boy, Nachiketa, visits the realm of Yama, the Lord of Death to seek knowledge of the eternal truths.
Koan (Japanese)	:	word or phrase creating a problem that cannot be solved by the intellect or pure reason or thought, but one which requires intuitive understanding, a leap of faith.
Kriya	:	root—*kri*, to act. an action being performed. Distinct from karma, which is a completed action.
Kriya Diksha	:	initiation into Kriya Yoga.
Kriya Yoga	:	practices that are aimed at purifying the body and the nervous system for ascendance to higher states of consciousness. Series of recharging exercises and meditation techniques

that lead to the ultimate liberation (realization) of the divine nature of the Self or soul.

Kumbh(Kumbha) : (i) literal meaning: vessel.

(ii) The Kumbh mela or festival is celebrated every twelve years at each of four sites, where according to legend, the elixir of life fell from the vessel carrying it.

(iii) The term Kumbh is also used to refer to a special spiritual gathering of sages.

Kundalini : literal meaning, the coiled one. The cosmic shakti or dormant potential that lies coiled in the body. When kundalini awakens in the body it moves up the central subtle channel piercing the chakras and initiating various yogic processes that bring about total purification and rejuvenation of the entire being.

Kutiya : dwelling place.

Lila : divine play of consciousness.

Maha : great, eternal.

Mahabharata : India's greatest epic poem, fifteen times longer than the Bible. The first written versions of it date back to the fifth or sixth century BC.

Mahamandalesh-war : title conferred on a respected sanyasi who heads a sect, region or religious order.

Mahant : spiritual leader, head of an ashram or sect.

Maharaj : literally, king, a term used to refer to a respected sage.

Mahatma : great soul.

Mahavtar : great incarnation of the divine.

Mandir : temple.

Mantra : root–*manas,* mind; *tra* to protect. Mantras are words or syllables that are recited during meditation practice to release the mind from unfocussed activity and prepare it for the state of illumination.

Mataji : an affectionate term meaning "mother", used for a guru or a holy woman.

Mauna : observance of spiritual silence.

Maya : the primal substance from which nature is formed. One of its qualities is form producing. However, while it produces form it also tends to veil the truth. When a mind starts to identify with the form instead of the underlying reality, it experiences a diminishing of intuitive and intellectual capacities. The truth hides behind this veil. Maya, therefore, is illusory but not an illusion.

Mithai : sweetmeat.

Mukti : liberation.

Muni : sage or saint.

Nachiketa (or Nachiketas) : literally *Na Chiketas,* the unperceived, the spirit or the flame that burns within. Nachiketa is the young seeker in the Kathopanishad who journeys to Yama, the lord of Death and seeks knowledge of the ultimate state of being, immortality and the Unmanifest.

Nirvana : state of liberation, beyond duality, where the atman merges in the paramatman. Ignorance and conflicting emotions cease and the atman attains freedom from compulsive rebirth in samsara.

Pandavas : descendants of Pandu, patronymic for five sons of Pandu, heroes of the Hindu epic *Mahabharata*.

Paramatman : p*aram*, beyond or transcendental; plus atman. Thus, the Supreme Soul.

Parikrama : circumambulation.

Parvati : literally, daughter of the Himalayas, eternal consort of Shiva.

Prakriti : source, original or material cause of anything, nature, the manifest universe.

Prana : the life force that pervades nature.

Pranam : to salute or bow in reverence.

Pranayama : breathing exercises, breath control practised in Yoga that regulates the strength and circulation of prana in the body.

Prasad : an offering made to the divine, which is then distributed to devotees with his blessings.

Pravachan : a religious discourse.

Purush : pure, unmanifested consciousness.

Quila : fort.

Ramayana : one of the great Hindu epics.

Renunciate : one who has relinquished attachment to objects, emotional states and actions.

Rishi : sage or saint.

Rudraksha : seeds from a tree known to be sacred to Shiva. Often strung as beads on a string and worn as a mala (necklace).

Sadhak	:	one who is on the spiritual path.
Sadhu	:	a monk, an ascetic.
Samadhi	:	root–*sam,* to put together. Complete consciousness. A state of consciousness where the yogi separates the astral and causal bodies and wanders in the Bramhand (the cosmic sphere). When a yogi is in a state of samadhi, his body appears lifeless and his thoughts assume a perfect balance. This is not a trance state but one of clear and undifferentiated awareness.
Sthal Samadhi	:	samadhi taken under ground.
Jal Samadhi	:	samadhi taken under water.
Samsara	:	objective world, sea of change, cycle of birth and death, characterised by suffering.
Samskaras	:	subtle impressions. All actions, whether mental, physical or verbal, leave subtle impressions on the mind. These lead us to action, which strengthens our samskaras and so on, leading to a never-ending cycle.
Sankalpa	:	will and determination towards a predetermined end, to make an event or circumstance or thing to manifest.
Sant	:	saint.
Sanyasi	:	ascetic. One who has forsaken the household life to seek knowledge (female equivalent sannyasini).
Sat/Satya/Satva	:	truth. Also harmony and purity.
Satvik	:	from *Satva,* or Satya, truth, harmony and purity.

Shakti : cosmic creative force. Also the aspect of kundalini which, when aroused, leads to positive spiritual awakening.

Shiva : a name for the all-pervasive supreme reality; also the third aspect of the Hindu trinity, symbolising the destructive aspect.

Shloka : a short verse.

Shraddha : faith.

Siddha : perfect, realised or enlightened being. One who has acquired siddhis.

Siddhi : spiritual powers that control self, others and the forces of nature.

Swayamvara : ceremonial occasion at which suitors are invited so a girl can choose her own groom.

Tandava : a dance form representing the forces of life and death. It is associated with Lord Shiva and is referred to as Ananda Tandava when it is performed in joy and Rudra Tandav when performed for the purpose of destruction.

Tantra : root–*tan*, to expand. A system of practices for achieving particular goals, awaken innate abilities and achieve union with the infinite. The meaning of the word extends in the context of weaving and expanding the fabric of life.

Tantrik : a practitioner of tantra.

Tapasya : penance, asceticism.

Tika : a mark placed on the forehead signifying commitment to a spiritual ideal.

Triloka : literally the three worlds, earth, heaven and the nether regions.

Triloka Tika : symbol of universal protection.

Trishul : a trident, symbol of Lord Shiva.

Upanishads : the end part of the Vedas, a collection of sacred texts. Root, *Upa*, under; *ni*, near and *sad*, sit. Sitting at the feet of an illumined master. The Upanishads reveal the accumulated wisdom of the sages, which show the path to ultimate knowledge of the Brahman.

Upma : South Indian preparation with semolina.

Vaikunth : the celestial abode associated with Vishnu.

Vairagya : renunciation, freedom from desire, detachment.

Vedas : root–*vid*, to know, therefore the revealed knowledge of the sages. The Hymns of the Vedas date back to perhaps 1500 BC and are the oldest religious scriptures known. The Vedas consist of four collections, Rig, Sama, Yajur and Atharva. The first part of the Vedas, the Karma Kanda, preserves ancient hymns, rituals and codes of conduct. The second part, the Jnana Kanda, contains the Upanishads, the sacred teachings.

Videhi : one who is in his subtle or light body, one who can materialise and dematerialise his body at will.

Yagna/yagya : ritual sacrifice of the Vedas.

Yama : the first mortal. Lord of the region of Death.

Yoga : union. The Path, which leads to the ultimate union, the Self merging with Universal Consciousness.

Yogi : one who travels on the Path. A practitioner of Yoga.